Remember when you chose a career in EMS. . . .
Do you sometimes have a hard time remembering why?

Medic Life: Creating Success in EMS is a valuable resource for all EMS professionals. Learn how to create your own success and build the EMS career you want.

Medic Life provides a step-by-step method to help you define your own success, clarify your purpose, launch a successful job campaign, create daily success, and work with your EMS organization.

Medic Life prepares you for a rewarding and fulfilling career in EMS.

Here's what some EMS professionals have to say about *Medic Life: Creating Success in EMS*. . . .

"It's about time somebody started to look at the human issues confronting the provider. To date, it seems that everything in print deals only with the people we care for. Providers have needs, too."

O. J. Doyle, President, Doyle Consulting, Board Member, EMS of Minnesota

"One of the greatest challenges in EMS is to give ourselves permission to evaluate and praise ourselves. This book goes a long way towards cultivating that self-praise and self-assessment."

Chip Boehm, RN, EMT-P, Training Coordinator, Maine EMS

"Recognizes EMS from the individual's perspective instead of from the system's as is often done."

Therese Specher, Director of Clinical Support Services, Life Link III

"I would use this text as prerequisite reading for traditional EMS programs."

David Miller, President, HealthSpan Transportation Services

"There are clear indications that more attention needs to be given to the needs of EMS professionals. Medic Life addresses those needs."

Steven Kanarian, EMT-P, ALS Special Assistant, New York City EMS

"This text will be invaluable to all enlightened EMS systems that recognize that good prehospital care begins before meeting patients and extends far beyond clinical medicine."

Kate Dernocoeur, Paramedic, Author of *Streetsense*

MEDIC LIFE

Creating Success in EMS

To. David,

thanks for all your encouragment

during this adventure.

Your Bro-

John

MEDIC LIFE

Creating Success in EMS

JOHN BECKNELL

A JEMS BOOK

 Mosby
Lifeline

St. Louis   Baltimore   Boston   Carlsbad   Chicago   Naples   New York   Philadelphia   Portland
London   Madrid   Mexico City   Singapore   Sydney   Tokyo   Toronto   Wiesbaden

Acquisitions Editor: Rina Steinhauer
Developmental Editor: Carole Anderson
Editorial Assistant: Melissa Blair

Library of Congress Cataloging-in-Publication Data
Becknell, John, 1956-
  Medic life : creating success in EMS / John Becknell.
      p.   cm.
    Includes bibliographical references.
    ISBN 0-8151-3046-5 (soft)
    1. Emergency medical services—Vocational guidance.   2. Emergency
medical technicians.   3. Becknell, John, 1956-   .   I. Title.
    [DNLM: 1. Emergency Medical Technicians.   2. Career Mobility.
3. Motivation.   W 21.5 B397m 1995]
    RA645.5.B43   1995
    362.1'8'023—dc20
    DNLM/DLC
    for Library of Congress   95-872
                                                                CIP

ISBN: 0-8151-3046-5
Book Code: 24768
Jems Product Code: JP0200

Jems Communications
A division of Mosby-Year Book, Inc.
P.O. Box 2789
Carlsbad, California 92018
(619) 431-9797

A JEMS BOOK

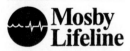

Dedicated to Publishing Excellence

A Times Mirror Company

Mosby-Year Book, Inc.
11830 Westline Industrial Drive
St. Louis, Missouri 63146

Publishing coordination and book production by
Laing Communications Inc., Redmond, Washington, and Edmonton, Alberta

Design and Production: Sandra J. Harner
Editorial Coordination: Christine Laing, Susan Bureau

Contents

To my sons, Joshua and Justin,
who have taught me life's
most important lessons in success.

Foreword

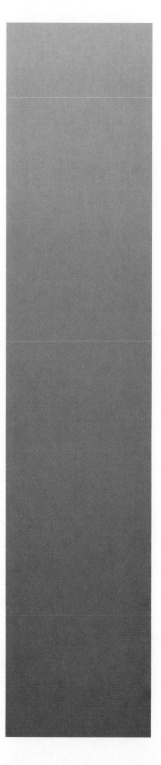

Success in emergency medical services. What is it? Is it possible? Can it be found? How will you know when you find it? These questions or others like them have plagued all of us who have chosen to pursue a career in this fast-paced, dynamic, incredibly stimulating field known as EMS.

We like working in this field. We think it would be terrific to find a way to spend the rest of our lives working in emergency medical services. But, while we want this career to work, we also constantly hear that EMS is a young person's occupation and that the average career in EMS lasts five years. We look at the ever-increasing requirements for maintaining the necessary knowledge and proficiency to be good in this field. We look at the physical and psychological risks associated with EMS. We look at the meager paycheck we receive at the end of the week. We wonder, frankly, if there is any way to make a life-long career in EMS work.

Is a long, successful career in EMS possible? The answer is an unequivocal yes. There are examples all around us in EMS, and more are turning up every day. All that is needed to achieve success in EMS is personal energy and initiative, as well as the tools to get the job done. You must provide the energy and initiative yourself, but John Becknell has assembled all of the tools for you—right here between the covers of this book.

I have had the privilege of enjoying a considerable amount of success in my personal career in EMS. Over a period of more than 20 years, I have gone from a rookie firefighter/EMT in the Anne Arundel County (Maryland) Fire Department to director of EMS for the State of Colorado to my current position as associate executive director with the American College of Emergency Physicians. The details would take up much more space than is available here, but the important point is that John Becknell has captured all of the key elements of my own career growth in this book. It is almost as if he were there watching as my career grew—one step at a time. I am sure that other readers who have enjoyed success in this business would agree that *Medic Life: Creating Success in EMS* must be read by anyone interested in an EMS career.

Medic Life starts with a basic definition of success. No, the author cannot define it for you; success is something that is deeply personal. However, the book does help you arrive at your personal definition. You are then led through a process of self-examination that starts with your self-esteem and self-confidence, two essential characteristics for success. The good news is that they can be developed, and *Medic Life* shows you how. You are encouraged to focus on your goals, develop a personal purpose, and constantly work at clarifying that purpose as you grow and develop.

Once you have your self-assessment in hand and a clear purpose in sight, John Becknell provides some practical guidance for finding a job, getting started in a new position, and seeking opportunities for career growth and development. There is an excellent chapter on keeping the "right" attitude in your daily work that will help anyone who has ever experienced frustration at the "system" around them. Practical suggestions on how to deal with management and how to become a productive team member focus on real-life situations that we have all faced.

Finally, Becknell deals with what he calls the "tough stuff." These are the things that put a real strain on our commitment to success—like the call that goes bad, system abuse, and lack of appreciation. The book also deals with the challenges to personal relationships that an EMS career can create. While divorce and destroyed friendships are common in EMS, they are not inevitable if you have the right tools and are willing to work at your relationships.

This book does more than just identify challenges; it gives practical, EMS-related strategies for you to use in your own life. Written in a friendly style, it is filled with practical information and exercises for you to complete. This is not just textbook theory; the author speaks as someone who has established a productive career and enjoyed success in EMS.

John Becknell and I are fortunate. We have had the extraordinary good fortune to enjoy careers in EMS that can only be described as love affairs. Our good fortune is out there and reachable for those who are willing to work at it. As the title of the book suggests, success does not just happen—it is created. Reading *Medic Life: Creating Success in EMS* is the first step in creating your own success in emergency medical services.

William R. Metcalf
January 1995

Preface

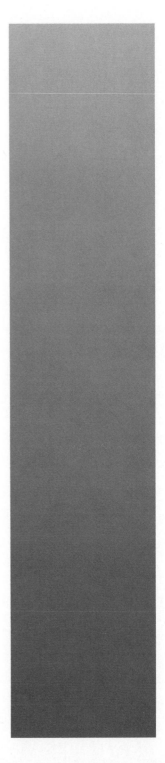

Medic Life: Creating Success in EMS is for everyone in EMS work, but it's not about emergency medicine and how to take care of patients—it's about you. Specifically, this book addresses how you can be successful while working as an EMT or paramedic (the term "medic" is used to apply to both). The book is full of practical help for shaping an EMS career that goes beyond just *doing things right,* to the life-giving practice of *doing the right thing*.

Medic Life addresses the basic human need to have meaning in our work lives. EMS work should not simply be labor. Our work should be an expression of who we are and our unique abilities. It should go beyond celebrating the lives we save and become an expression of how valuable our own lives can be.

In 1975, I began my work as an EMT ambulance attendant. It was a heady time for this new concept called EMS. The Vietnam War was over, Johnny and Roy were calling Rampart from everyone's living room, and the government was promoting the concept with generous amounts of money, training, and equipment. Like so many other eager young people of that time, I wanted to do something that mattered. I signed up for the ride, and what a ride it was. In those early days, we loved our patches, our scissor holsters, our exactly performed CPR, and the screaming federal sirens on our Cadillacs. No one cared much about EMS as a career. No one talked about success. Our needs were simple. We wanted people to stop calling us "ambulance drivers," and we wanted another exciting call.

Time passed, and EMS became much more than a young person's adventure. I hung around, and it slowly turned into a career. I liked the idea of helping people, the idea of doing something relevant, and the unpredictable working environment. But as EMS became more of a career, it also became a job, and after awhile I didn't feel very successful. In fact, the longer I stayed in EMS, the more frustrated I became.

I thought the problem was my position, so I tried changing jobs. I tried a busier service, I tried management and education positions, I tried being a flight medic, and I even took my EMS work overseas to teach and practice in a foreign culture. By most people's standards, I was successful, but in my own mind, I often felt a lot like that "ambulance driver." Along the way I had become many things—the workaholic, the victim, the self-denying rescuer, the unappreciated civil servant, and the bitter hero for whom no yellow ribbons had been hung. For some reason, I could not find the success or satisfaction I wanted.

At least I wasn't alone. Many of my EMS colleagues expressed the same theme of great expectations and frustrating payoffs. I finally concluded that such disappointment was just part of the EMS experience. So, after a dozen years of service, I started planning to leave.

In an effort to prepare myself for leaving EMS, I did two things. First, I began a vigorous study of successful people. I read stacks of self-help books on creating success, and I talked with people who appeared to be successful and happy in their work and life. Second, I began to pay attention to what really mattered to me as a street medic. Since I was leaving, I started focusing on the things that were valuable to me. I had seen many people leave EMS bitter and frustrated, and I vowed to go out smiling. To that end, I quit worrying about things I couldn't change. I quit complaining about management, partners, and paychecks and, instead, focused on what brought me satisfaction and joy in the work. I started having fun again. As I did these two things, something unexpected began to happen. I began to learn some powerful lessons about success.

I learned that, above all else in rescue work, I have to pay attention to myself and take good care of me. People in helping professions often become victims themselves. They give endlessly to others and neglect themselves while expecting a big payoff "someday." But the reward for self-neglect never comes, and eventually they are used up and left feeling cynical and abused. This is a destructive cycle rooted in poor self-esteem. When I started treating myself with the same sort of reverence and respect I gave my patients, my perspective changed. Instead of saving the world, I began to save myself.

I learned that I alone am responsible for my career happiness. It's easy to expect someone else to make me happy. It's easy to blame the job, management, and the state of EMS for my lack of happiness. But I am in the driver's seat. I am not captive to my external circumstances. Success and happiness are within my control.

I also learned that I need to have a sense of purpose in my work. If I believe my EMS work is just another job—it is. In order for work to be extraordinary, I need to have a clear picture of what it looks like and how it relates to me, my history, my dreams, and my values. At first, the thought of focusing on what I really wanted seemed selfish and myopic, but once I began to uncover

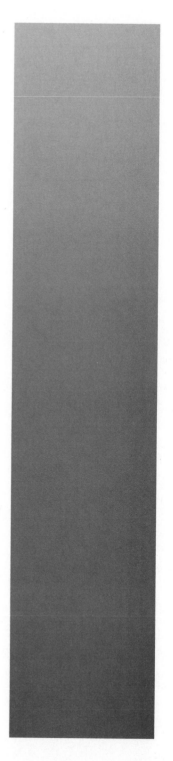

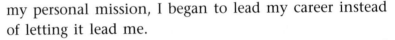

my personal mission, I began to lead my career instead of letting it lead me.

Further, I learned that I truly need others. I need management, my fellow workers, my family, and even my patients. But I had to learn to relate to each apart from the rescue paradigm.

As I applied these learnings, things began to change. I found myself enjoying my shifts more than ever before. Regardless of the current state of the organization, management, or even the economy, I was creating personal success. By applying these lessons, I began to find the satisfaction I had been looking for. I became less concerned about things I could not change. I focused on those unique moments that encompass the wonderful mysteries of humanity, love, service, and life itself.

I wrote *Medic Life* for a number of reasons. First, I wanted to validate that EMS can indeed be rich and fulfilling work. Second, I wanted to validate that the frustrations and craziness many EMS workers feel are real and not just personal flaws. I wanted to show that burnout is not the automatic end to working in EMS. Third, I wrote *Medic Life* in the hopes that I might leave the field a little better for those who follow. Should either of my two sons choose to work in EMS, I want them to benefit from my experience and perhaps step over a few holes I fell into. Finally, I wrote *Medic Life* to learn. It has been said that we teach what we most need to learn. I am still learning as I share these principles with you. Success is not a grand destination somewhere in the future. It is an everyday habit that requires continual learning.

Oh, yes, I have not left EMS. I am writing this at a small desk in an ambulance station as I await calls. While there are many things to do in EMS, there is nothing quite like being a field medic. It is here that I find the most joy.

The American sage Joseph Campbell once said, "A hero is someone who has given one's life to something bigger than oneself." EMS is indeed bigger than we are. It is much more than medical science on wheels or helping others. It is an adventure full of heroic possibilities and unpredictable dangers. My hope is that this book will reawaken your dreams and your passion for something bigger. I hope it will stimulate you to take some action and move from reactive waiting to proactive creation of lasting success. Don't settle for anything less.

John Michael Becknell

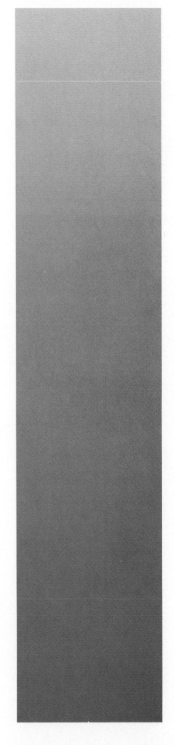

Author's Acknowledgments

Writing a book, like a good rescue call, is always more than a solo effort. I owe much to my paramedic partners, who over the last year continually encouraged me to write, patiently read the chapters, argued about my ideas, and shared their lives and stories with me.

I am very grateful to Carole Anderson, one of the finest editors in EMS, for her exceptional editing of the book, her encouraging phone calls, generous friendship, and understanding ear. Without her help, this book would have been much less.

A special thank you to Melissa Blair, David Page, Steve Kanarian, David Miller, and all of the others who read and commented on the work in progress.

The whole idea of expressing myself through writing is wrapped up in the nurturing support of my brother, Thomas Becknell, who has always believed in my ability to do great things.

Finally, in the middle of this project when I often felt like giving up, a quiet, reassuring voice continually reminded me, even on the darkest nights, that I was loved—thanks, Joyce.

Publisher's Acknowledgments

The publisher wishes to thank the following individuals for their time and input as reviewers of this book:

Chip Boehm, RN, EMT-P
Training Coordinator
Maine EMS
Falmouth, Maine

Kate Dernocoeur, EMT-P
Speaker, Writer
Team Dernocoeur
Grand Rapids, Michigan

Jeff Lucia, NREMT-P
Technical Editor
JEMS
Ventura, California

1 Defining Success

Men were born to succeed, not to fail.

—Henry David Thoreau

Welcome to Emergency Medical Services. There is something powerfully attractive about this work. The emergency tones sound, the dispatcher calls out the number of your rig, and suddenly you're responding to an auto accident. The radio crackles as your truck weaves through traffic, and the voice of a police officer announces that she has multiple victims and needs an extrication tool. Your pulse quickens as you switch the siren from wail to yelp.

People usually don't choose EMS work on a whim; they are irresistibly drawn to it. As one rescuer described it, "I came to EMS for the excitement of the work and the chance to really help people."

Another said, "I've always been drawn to action. I like to be where things are happening."

Still another explained, "I was working in a retail job and was very unhappy. One day, I watched some paramedics taking care of a woman at a car wreck, and I knew I wanted to do something that mattered to people. I

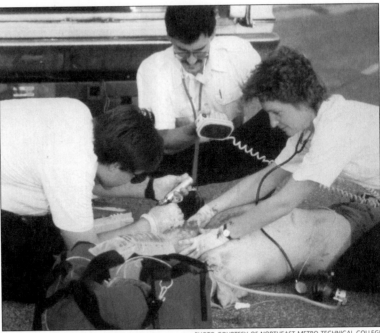

PHOTO COURTESY OF NORTHEAST METRO TECHNICAL COLLEGE

wanted to be involved in work that made a difference—no matter how small that difference was." Whether it's the excitement, the intensity, or the chance to help others, EMS offers many opportunities for extraordinary work.

Unlike a paper-shuffling job in a cushy, air-conditioned office, emergency response is full of noise, action, and adventure. All elements of an emergency—the pager tones, the lights and sirens, the fast pace, the crackle of the radio, the teamwork, and the lives at risk—create an intense, highly charged work environment. Even on a slow day, one knows the next moment could bring a heart-pounding call to the very edge of life and death. Little is predictable and every day brings unlimited possibilities.

But beyond the excitement, EMS offers work that is full of meaning and purpose. When a call comes for an unresponsive child trapped in a sewer pipe, there is no question the rescuer is needed and is making a valuable contribution to the community. Few jobs compare

EMS offers work that is full of meaning and purpose.

to the relevance of rushing to help someone who is in serious need.

Even more, EMS is full of the drama of human life. It is a journey into the homes and back alleys of peoples' lives. Emergencies—and non-emergencies—can be a limitless social education, and the potential for new experiences is only a pager tone away. Even non-EMS people are captured by the drama. "What's it like?" they ask. They want to hear about rescues and watch them replayed on television.

Despite all EMS promises, many people don't find the satisfaction and fulfillment they expected. Evidence of this is seen among the many veteran EMS workers who are frustrated and disillusioned.

Kathy, a paramedic for several years in Arizona, described her experience this way: "After going to college for several years to be a physical therapist, I switched to EMS and became a medic. The immediate nature of the work and everything about it seemed to be just what I was looking for. I fell in love with work. I looked forward to my shifts, and I was proud to tell everyone I was a medic. But now that I've been doing it for a few years, I'm disappointed. I haven't found what I was looking for. I'm not sure I can even explain why, but I just know I'm not happy. I'm not getting much out of the work anymore."

Kathy is not alone. Many EMS workers express similar feelings of frustration and lack of fulfillment. And surprisingly, it's not just crusty old veterans who feel this way; disillusionment can rear its head at any stage of an EMS career.

When I first began working in EMS, I expected every day to be a breathtaking experience. I envisioned responding to one great call after another. I wasn't prepared for the more routine part of the job—the waiting around and the endless demands of being in a service job. Before long,

> Emergencies, as well as non-emergencies, can be a limitless social education, and the potential for new experiences is only a pager tone away.

I began to question my decision to work in EMS and eventually became extremely frustrated and disgruntled.

How could this happen? How could such a potentially rewarding job become so maddeningly monotonous? There are many reasons, including the difficult nature of the work, the newness and ongoing development of EMS as a career field, the many ways in which EMS workers are used and abused by EMS organizations, and the huge changes affecting the field as healthcare reform takes shape. Yet, an even bigger reason is one that lies within the workers themselves.

Many EMS workers mistakenly think they will find the great work experience they want by simply completing their training and climbing into an ambulance. For a while, the excitement will sustain them, but eventually, the thrill of emergencies will not be enough. They will also learn that the last letter in EMS stands for *service,* and service to other human beings can often take much more from us than it gives back.

So, is EMS work an empty promise? Is it like so many new cars, vacations, and barroom romances—a lot of hype and no substance? While it may seem that way, a growing number of EMS workers are discovering that they *can* have a fulfilling and rewarding EMS experience. The secret is in recognizing that achieving a sense of success in EMS takes more than just passing a skills test and jumping on an ambulance. It requires more than just responding quickly to exciting calls. Success in EMS is something you *create* by applying very specific principles and skills.

Imagine being the first unit in on a real grinder. The scene is chaotic and tense. The victims are moaning in pain, and the bystanders are yelling for you to do something. Merely being there with a truck full of equipment and medical gadgets will not give you control of the scene or help your patients. You'll get control of the situation and help the victims by using the principles and skills you have studied, practiced, and perfected during your training.

The same is true for creating success in your career. You need to know and use the principles and skills of success. While not a part of your EMT or paramedic curriculum, skills for success can be learned and practiced in much the same way you learned to backboard, triage, and write a report. Before we talk about these principles and skills, let's first explore the concept of success and its relationship to EMS.

What Is Success?

The word "success" is not usually applied to emergency work. In our society, it's most often used to describe achievement in the areas of money, power, prestige, and fame. When people talk about being successful, they are

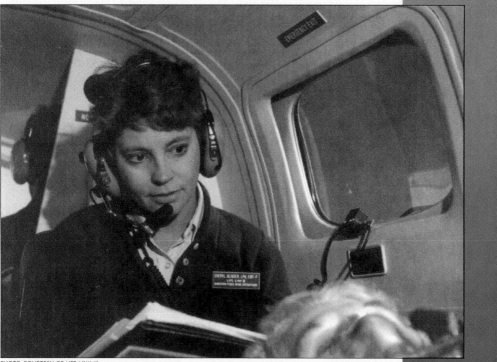

Success/sək sĕs/ n. favorable outcome, accomplishment of what was aimed at, attainment of wealth or fame or position; thing or person that turns out well; outcome.

—*Oxford Dictionary of Current English*

The most important definer of your success is you.

usually referring to a recognized level of achievement. Athletes are successful if they win a certain competition. Musicians are successful if they sell a certain number of records. Actors are successful if they star in a big production. Business people are successful if they make a certain amount of money.

In EMS, we may consider ourselves successful when a certain level of training is completed or a desirable job is found, or even when a rescue attempt leads to a positive result. Most of us don't enter the field looking for special recognition or societal rewards. Yet, in choosing EMS, we are hoping for *something*. Perhaps it's not money, power, or fame, but we are looking for some kind of reward or satisfaction that meets our needs. We may want daily work that's not boring, or the chance to help people, or the good feelings that come from knowing we've done a great job in a stressful situation.

The word success means to have a favorable outcome. The important question is, who defines what is favorable? Society can define it, your co-workers can define it, or you can define it. You may be influenced by many different definitions, but the most important definer of your success is you.

So, what does success in EMS mean? To truly be successful means experiencing what you consider to be a

Consider this alternate definition of success:
After the famous Indian leader Mahatma Gandhi died, a photograph was taken of all his earthly possessions: a pair of spectacles, a pair of sandals, a few simple garments, a spinning wheel, and a book. Yet Gandhi is often considered one of the world's most successful men. His riches were much more than material.

favorable outcome, satisfying and pleasing yourself. Too often in work and life, people embark on the dubious task of fulfilling other people's expectations without giving much regard to their own. This is particularly true of EMS workers. They always seem to be taking care of someone else, pleasing someone else, or meeting another's expectations. But such efforts do not produce real personal success. History books are full of stories of people who have been wildly successful at pleasing others, often achieving great heights, but failing miserably at pleasing themselves.

When we talk about success in this book, we're talking about creating success in *your* eyes. The important thing is finding a favorable outcome that pleases *you*. What do *you* want from EMS work? How can *you* create the sort of experience that will make you glad you entered this field? So much of EMS and its training is focused on other people that the individual EMS worker often loses sight of what he wants from the experience. In this book, we want to change the focus from everyone else to you. What do *you* really want from this work, and what do *you* want as your reward?

The ideas presented here are based on several assumptions. First, choosing EMS work is more than a selfless act; there is something to be gained from it. Second, work in general should be fulfilling and satisfying for the person doing it; work does not have to be labor. Third, burnout and frustration need not be the outcome of EMS work. You can create a successful EMS experience while enjoying daily work that continues to be exciting, gratifying, and even joyful for years to come.

So whether you are an old hand at EMS or a newcomer, this book is for you. Success is something you can begin creating at any time—it's never too late. In fact, if you've been in EMS for a while, you'll better understand many of the principles and ideas discussed here.

"Success, if it is to be meaningful, must be a personal thing. It varies from individual to individual as personality varies; indeed, it springs from the very depths where personality itself arises, and often it takes insightful probing to find out for ourselves what our own ideas of success actually are."
—Howard Whitman

You can create a successful EMS experience while enjoying daily work that continues to be exciting.

"Two roads diverged in a wood, and I—I took the one less traveled by, and that has made all the difference."

—From Robert Frost's "The Road Not Taken"

On the other hand, if you're new to EMS, you'll be exposed to many things that can help you create success from the very start. Regardless of where you are in your career, beginning to create success in EMS will have an effect on your entire life. As you will see, many of the principles we discuss in relationship to EMS will apply to other areas of your life.

More About Success

To better understand how you can create a favorable outcome for yourself in EMS, let's take a closer look at success and its most important principle. A good way to think of success is to imagine that it is a road and that you are building it. As the sole builder, you have complete freedom to make the road any way you want. It can be a big, broad highway or a small, winding path. Your road can be smooth and paved, or it can be rough and full of stones and potholes. It's your road, so you can choose the direction it will go. Your road can race through large cities, meander through quiet meadows, or climb high vistas overlooking picturesque valleys.

Furthermore, because you are building the road, you can change its direction any time you wish. You can make a sharp left turn and loop back to where you started, or perhaps, like the poet Robert Frost suggested, you can angle off into a less traveled part of the woods. What's exciting about building this road is that you are totally in charge. You can even sit down and rest, or you can decide not to build a road at all. The choice is totally yours.

Notice we've compared success to a road, not a destination. People often make the mistake of seeing success as a distant goal or destination. They say, "I'll be successful when I've achieved that promotion," or "I'll be successful when I'm out of debt and have so much money in the bank." But success is not a destination. It's a journey. Success in EMS is a process that begins the moment

Success is not a destination. It's a journey.

you define the outcome you desire. The problem is, most people doubt their ability to build the road to success.

The Great Lie

Believing that we create our own success is a tough pill to swallow. In this TV and lottery world of superstars, we've been infected with the Great Lie, which says success is all about breaks, good luck, being in the right place at the right time, or having exceptional talent. The Great Lie tells us that life is determined by the things that happen to us. It says that with only minor exceptions, we have to accept life just as it is, that we cannot really change things. It whispers, "You're just a product of your upbringing, heritage, and circumstances—you can't change anything." It taunts us with long-shot hopes such as, "Maybe you'll win the lottery," or "Perhaps someone will discover you one day and make you famous." This lie causes many people to limit themselves, settle for less, not consider the possibilities, and stand by, simply waiting for another throw of the dice.

A big champion of the Great Lie was Sigmund Freud. Freud was the psychiatrist who taught that we are merely the products of our genetic makeup, upbringing, and environment. He taught that we can do very little to change the natural course of our lives and that life is determined by things beyond our control. His theory became known as determinism.

Determinism is reflected throughout our society in everyday conversations. People say things such as, "I can't help it. . . ," "If only I had. . . ," "My parents were. . . ," or "I just have to accept. . . ."

And I frequently hear determinism reflected in EMS circles when people say, "I can't get the job I want. . . ," "My boss won't let me. . . ," "I'm just lucky. . . ," and "Oh well, shit happens." Determinism is the philosophy that allows people to blame the rest of the world for their

> *"Success is simply a matter of luck. Ask any failure."*
> —Earl Wilson

> *"If you keep on saying things are going to be bad, you have a good chance of being a prophet."*
> —Isaac Bashevis Singer

> *"I know of no more encouraging fact than the unquestionable ability of man to elevate his life by conscious endeavor."*
>
> —Henry David Thoreau

lack of success. Determinists can duck responsibility for the course of their lives by blaming their childhood, their current financial problems, their lack of talent, or a streak of bad luck. The Great Lie of determinism says success in life is beyond your control.

Beyond the Great Lie

Interestingly, determinism emerged largely from the study of people with serious mental problems. When studying people who have lived exciting, fulfilling, and meaningful lives, determinism doesn't hold up. In fact, the opposite is true. People create success in spite of failures, handicaps, disappointments, and even severe limitations.

One of the most startling challenges to Freud's determinism comes from one of his students, another psychiatrist named Viktor Frankl. Frankl studied with Freud in Vienna, Austria, and was a follower of his ideas. During World War II, the Nazis sent Frankl to a concentration camp. His wife, family, and many of his friends were put to death. Frankl was stripped of everything he had and was left in the prison camp to perform slave labor with hundreds of other men.

Viktor E. Frankl is a professor of neurology and psychiatry at the University of Vienna Medical School and is a distinguished professor of logotherapy at the United States International University. He is the founder of what has come to be called the Third Viennese School of Psychotherapy (after Freud's psychoanalysis and Adler's individual psychology), the school of logotherapy, or meaning therapy.

During World War II, Dr. Frankl spent three years at Auschwitz, Dachau, and other concentration camps. You can read the moving account of his experience and his powerful conclusions in his book, *Man's Search for Meaning.*

In his book, *Man's Search for Meaning*, Frankl tells about the horrors of the concentration camp, where life indeed seemed determined by the awful circumstances he endured. One day, though, while being used for painful medical experimentation, Frankl made a startling discovery: No matter what the Nazis did to him, he still had the freedom to choose how he would respond. He discovered that even though his physical circumstances were severely restricted, his life was not totally determined, and he was not completely helpless. He had choices. Would he give up? Would he despair? Would he try to survive a bit longer? Would he continue to have hope? He realized he could determine many things and that no matter what was happening around him—and even to him—he still had the freedom to choose.

Frankl found that Freud had been wrong. Life is not just a sum of circumstances, environment, and heritage. This discovery had a profound effect on his outlook in prison camp. He found reasons to be hopeful, as well as the strength not only to survive, but to become a powerful help to his fellow prisoners. Even in prison and despite his terrible circumstances, Frankl created a road to success. After the war, he went on to found an important school of thought based on the principle that people do have a powerful influence over their destiny.

Accepting that you can make a difference in your life is the most important principle in creating your success in EMS. No matter what your circumstances, you will always be the most important influence in your work and your life. No matter what disadvantages you face, you can create the favorable outcome you want. Your success is not a stroke of luck; it depends on you taking responsibility for your life and creating what you really want. You will always be the most powerful force in creating your road to success.

Success in EMS does not begin with finding a great

> *"Many people wait for something to happen or someone to take care of them. But people who end up with the good jobs are the proactive ones who are solutions to problems, not problems themselves, who seize the initiative to do whatever is necessary, consistent with correct principles, to get the job done."*
>
> —Stephen Covey

You will always be the most powerful force in creating your road to success.

job, participating in a dramatic save, or responding to an exciting call. Success begins with the recognition that *you* create the outcome you want. The real adventure of EMS work comes from the very personal act of creating your success and accepting that you can have the experience that originally attracted you to this exciting field.

The balance of this book will teach you the skills and principles for creating your road to success. Starting with your core attitudes about yourself, you will learn how to define your success, find the job you want, create daily success, work with your EMS organization, find opportunities in tough stuff, and plan for the future.

Hidden Riches

Creating success is not easy. The skills and principles presented in this book demand work, practice, and personal honesty. When you begin to take an active role in creating success in your work, other aspects of your life may be affected. Changing old behaviors and attitudes can be uncomfortable, much like an uneasy journey into a strange land. But the rewards will be great. As Helen Keller once said, "Life is either a daring adventure, or it is nothing at all." The most difficult things in life can also be the most satisfying.

Few people come to EMS with the idea of making a lot of money, yet there are many hidden riches in this work. You have the chance to observe life at both its beginning and end. You are continually reminded of the passing of time and the importance of living each day to its fullest. Occasionally, you have the rare and priceless opportunity to save someone's life.

Yet, the real riches of your work will not be found in an accident or a good call. True satisfaction and fulfillment will evolve as you become an active participant in creating your own success. Happiness in work and life is not a result of some extraordinary event or coincidence;

it comes from knowing what you really want and creating your own favorable outcome.

Summary

- ✔ EMS is a great place to find a fulfilling and meaningful work experience.
- ✔ Many EMS workers don't find the experience they had hoped for.
- ✔ Creating success in EMS isn't automatic. It requires the application of special principles and skills.
- ✔ Success in EMS means creating a favorable experience or outcome in your eyes.
- ✔ Success must be defined and created by you.
- ✔ Creating success is a process, not a destination.
- ✔ Most people doubt their ability to create their own success.
- ✔ History shows that people are not a product of circumstance and are not bound by their circumstances.
- ✔ EMS holds many hidden riches for people who are willing to create their success.

Suggested Reading

Do It!, by John-Roger and Peter McWilliams (Prelude Press, Los Angeles, 1991). A fun and encouraging book about getting started in creating your success. This book is for people who don't read much. It's designed so that you can pick it up and get something worthwhile in just a moment or two of reading.

Man's Search for Meaning, by Viktor E. Frankl (Washington Square Press, New York, 1985). This is Viktor Frankl's

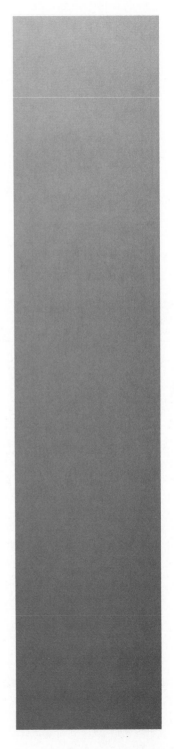

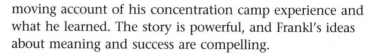

moving account of his concentration camp experience and what he learned. The story is powerful, and Frankl's ideas about meaning and success are compelling.

Og Mandino's University of Success, by Og Mandino (Bantam, New York, 1982). Og Mandino is one of the world's most widely read success writers. In this collection, he brings together some of the best of success literature. This book remains in print for a good reason—it works. If you read one selection per day, it will have a big impact on your life.

True Success: A New Philosophy of Excellence, by Thomas Morris, PhD (Grosset/Putnam Books, New York, 1994). Thomas Morris takes a straightforward and practical approach to success that goes beyond motivational material. He delves into what makes an ordinary person truly successful.

Wishcraft: How to Get What You Really Want, by Barbara Sher (Ballantine Books, New York, 1983). Using her own experience as testimony, Barbara Sher shows you how to begin turning dreams into reality. She shares her common-sense perspective and is full of encouragement.

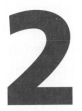

2

Honoring Yourself

Happiness and success in life do not depend upon our circumstances but on ourselves.

—Sir John Lubbock

During the glory years of the Green Bay Packers, legendary coach Vince Lombardi had the unique ability to focus his team on what was really important. During one particularly difficult game, he gathered his team in the locker room for a talk during half-time. As the players sat huddled and became quiet, Lombardi held up a football and said, "Gentlemen, it's time to get back to basics. This is a football." In EMS, success begins with the basics. You—and how you regard yourself—are the foundation of your success.

Consider some of the things you will have to accomplish before you can be successful in EMS. First, you will need to successfully complete a training program and pass a certification test. Next, you will need to negotiate the uneven terrain of the EMS job market. Once working, you will need to be able to apply your skills to help people

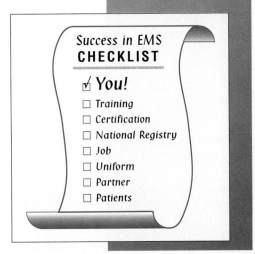

Success in EMS
CHECKLIST

☑ **You!**
☐ *Training*
☐ *Certification*
☐ *National Registry*
☐ *Job*
☐ *Uniform*
☐ *Partner*
☐ *Patients*

> *"Self-confidence is the first requisite for great undertakings."*
>
> —Samuel Johnson

in desperate situations and to manage frantic and chaotic emergency situations.

Yet, not all of the work will be so dramatic. You'll quickly discover that much of EMS is routine and humbling. You will learn about patience. On many of your calls, you will need the skills of a diplomat as you work with all kinds of people—with very different opinions of what should be happening—in high-stress situations. You will endure doctors who do not listen, managers who complicate your work, and patients you can't please. But there is hope: All of these situations can be less trying if you believe in yourself and your ability to succeed.

Success and Self-Esteem

When we talk about believing in ourselves, we're really talking about self-esteem. Self-esteem is the psychological term used to describe the way we think about ourselves. To be more precise, self-esteem is the confidence we have in our ability to cope with life and its challenges, coupled with the faith we have in our right to be happy.

Dr. Nathaniel Branden, one of the nation's leading experts on self-esteem and work, says, "Self-esteem is the key to success or failure." In EMS, just as in life, self-esteem is basic to everything. Skills, endurance, leadership, coping, relationships, and satisfaction are all affected by how we think of ourselves.

Most EMS workers appear to do well in the area of confidence; they learn to look and act confident with their emergency skills. They manage emergencies in a cool and calm manner. But having an exterior of confidence is not necessarily a sign of good self-esteem. The real test of self-esteem comes when we confront something that questions our actions and intentions and what we stand for.

A few years ago, I went on a call for a patient who was having respiratory distress. When my partner and I arrived, we found a man who was bleeding into his upper

> **"Self-esteem is the key to success or failure."**

airway. While the man was coughing, something had torn loose in his throat, and he was choking on his own blood. With my partner's help, I quickly began suctioning the man, but the blood was coming faster than it could be cleared away. I hesitated to intubate the man for fear of causing further bleeding, so I positioned him on his side to help the blood drain as we took off on the fifteen-minute ride to the hospital.

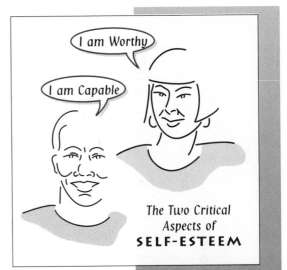

The Two Critical Aspects of
SELF-ESTEEM

I continued to suction and give oxygen, but it was not enough; I could see that the man was becoming cyanotic. I began to bag him and rolled him onto his back. After a few rapid ventilations, I attempted to intubate, but as I dipped in with the laryngoscope, the flow of blood blocked my view. I could see nothing. I suctioned the man, hyperventilated, and then attempted again—with no success. As I bagged him, I could feel his lungs becoming tighter and tighter. It was a desperate situation, but I could think of nothing else to try.

When we arrived at the hospital, the ED doctor had a difficult time placing the tube. He finally shoved it into place after numerous attempts, but it was too late. The man arrested several minutes later and was eventually pronounced dead.

As my partner and I were leaving, I overheard the doctor suggesting that my attempts at field intubation had made the problem worse. I was flushed with self-denunciation. I doubted what I had done. Why hadn't I been able to get that tube? Had I really done the wrong thing? Was I responsible for the man's death? I went home feeling terrible—not so much because of the man's death, but because I doubted myself. When confronted with a sudden and dramatic death, it's easy to doubt oneself.

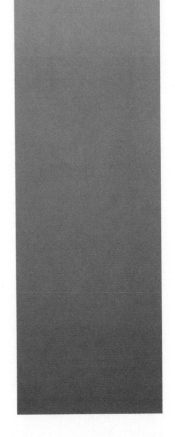

> *"There is no value judgment more important to man—no factor more decisive in his psychological development and motivation—than the estimate he passes on himself."*
>
> —Nathaniel Branden

If we do not like ourselves or believe in our ability to succeed, we cannot be successful.

Self-doubt is an awful emotion. No matter how exciting or rewarding work is, if we doubt ourselves, the joy and personal reward are diminished. This is true beyond the emergency call and in every aspect of our lives. When confronted with something difficult, the depth and quality of our self-esteem are tested. Deep inside, if we do not like ourselves or believe in our ability to succeed, we cannot be successful.

Underneath your EMS uniform, beyond the cool, external professional, how do you think of yourself? Are you confident in your actions and intentions? Do you believe in yourself? Do you like yourself?

Low self-esteem often remains hidden until we are confronted with a difficult situation, like the one described above. The following assessment will give you a glimpse of how you think and feel about yourself.

Try This:

Take a few minutes to complete the following assessment of your self-esteem. Using the simple point scoring, determine how much you agree or disagree with each statement (This exercise is for your eyes only, so be as honest as you can.). Add up the total score.

1 point—Strongly disagree with the statement.

2 points—Disagree with the statement.

3 points—Neutral about the statement; neither agree nor disagree.

4 points—Agree with the statement.

5 points—Strongly agree with the statement.

1. *I like myself.*	*1 2 3 4 5*
2. *I am competent.*	*1 2 3 4 5*
3. *I manage difficult life situations effectively.*	*1 2 3 4 5*
4. *I enjoy my own company.*	*1 2 3 4 5*

5. *People listen to my suggestions.*   *1 2 3 4 5*

6. *I am successful.*   *1 2 3 4 5*

7. *I trust my own judgment.*   *1 2 3 4 5*

8. *People like being with me.*   *1 2 3 4 5*

9. *I am not a failure.*   *1 2 3 4 5*

10. *In my social circle, people seek my company.*   *1 2 3 4 5*

11. *I have good ideas.*   *1 2 3 4 5*

12. *I am an attractive person.*   *1 2 3 4 5*

13. *I am a good friend to others.*   *1 2 3 4 5*

14. *I am proud of the things I do.*   *1 2 3 4 5*

   Total score   _____

The objective of this assessment is for you to evaluate your self-concept and assess whether your self-esteem is low or high. The maximum score you could have is 70 points; the higher your numbers, the higher your self-esteem. There are no typical scores and certainly no right or wrong answers, but if you think your self-esteem needs some boosting, there are several excellent books listed at the end of this chapter that can help.

Finding Self-Esteem in EMS

No matter how we score in self-esteem, we often look for ways to improve our self-confidence and opinion of ourselves. Many of us turn to work, relationships, accomplishments, and material things in an effort to feel and think better about ourselves. We often expect EMS to build our self-esteem.

In a recent discussion with a group of forty paramedic students about EMS and its effects on self-esteem, many of the participants said they strongly believed that EMS would improve their self-esteem. One woman who was working as an EMT told of going on a call for a 5-year-old boy who had been mauled by a dog. The child had

"The reason you cannot earn your worth is because you are already worthy. All you can do is accept what is already yours."

—Carmen Renee Berry

severe lacerations on his face and arms. The woman had been able not only to treat the wounds, but to provide assurance and comfort for both the child and his mother on the way to the hospital. "It was a terrible injury," the woman explained, "but in helping the child and mother, I felt great about myself and the work I was doing."

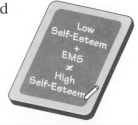

A Vitally Important Equation to Remember in EMS Work

Another student said EMS workers were well-respected in the small town where he worked. When he wore his uniform, people looked up to him and admired the work he did. He said he was proud to be in EMS and thought it contributed much to his self-esteem.

Another student spoke about becoming proficient in EMS. "My confidence has really grown since I've realized I can learn skills and become good at them," he said. "Becoming proficient in my cardiac arrest skills is a great feeling."

Yet another student told the story of being called to an old farmhouse where an elderly man had died during the night. "There was nothing we could do for the man," the student said, "so I went into the kitchen and sat down with the wife. At first I didn't know what to say, so I just started talking to her about what had happened. After a while, she began talking about her husband. She told me all about their life together. I listened, and we both cried. When we finally left, the woman gave me a big hug and said I had helped a lot."

All of these students described some of the great experiences of EMS, but playing the devil's advocate, I challenged their assertions that EMS builds self-esteem. I agreed that indeed, there are confidence-building experiences in EMS, but I also pointed out that for every positive experience there is a negative experience.

EMS can provide confidence-building experiences, but it is not a reliable builder of self-esteem.

Self-esteem is built from the inside out.

Often, your work will not be appreciated even by the people you are trying to help. You will be criticized on calls when something goes wrong, and frequently you will leave a patient not knowing if you really made a difference. There will be times when you want to help people but they are beyond even the best of your skills. There will be times when managers, doctors, nurses, and other responders appear oblivious to your efforts and show no signs of valuing your work.

The important point is this: EMS can provide confidence-building experiences, but it is not a reliable builder of self-esteem. The real evidence of this is seen in veteran EMS workers; if EMS were a great place to build self-esteem, the senior ranks would be filled with people bursting with positive views of themselves. But EMS is no different from any other job or life situation when it comes to self-esteem. Jobs, relationships, money, fame, and circumstances are not reliable builders of self-esteem. Self-esteem is built from the inside out.

Honoring Yourself

In EMS, we take care of patients, family, and other rescuers. In fact, because everything in EMS seems to focus on caring for others, many rescuers are uncomfort-

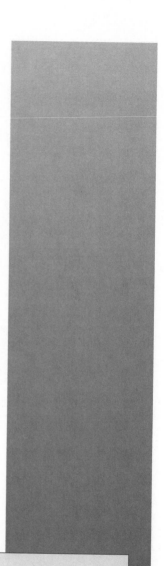

Honoring Yourself Is Not Narcissism

Narcissus is a character from Greek mythology who was pursued by many lovers. His haughty rejection of all of them, including the beautiful nymph Echo, led the gods to condemn him to a life of looking at himself in the reflection of a pond. For days he admired himself until he wasted away and died. The story illustrates the danger of self-absorption. Honoring yourself is not about falsely inflating your ego but about honestly acknowledging your value, capability, and worth.

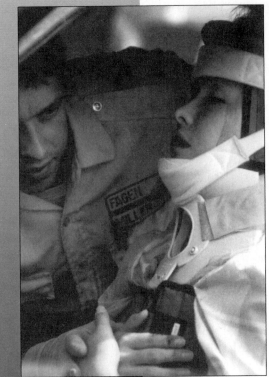

PHOTO BY MICHAEL KOWAL

able caring for themselves. Indeed, some of the most unpopular characters in any EMS community are those who talk about themselves, boast about their heroic feats, and arrogantly look down on others.

But to create success through healthy self-esteem, you must first honor yourself. This is not to suggest that you should adopt a conceited, self-serving, narcissistic attitude. Honoring yourself means acknowledging your worth and value with an attitude that says, *"My life is valuable and worthy and is the most important life I will ever care for."*

Consider one of the basic assumptions of people who work in EMS: We assume all life has value. Without considering who a patient is, what his social status is, or even the person's ability to pay, we respond to the scene of an emergency, sometimes risking our lives to save a stranger simply because we believe life has value. Therefore, if everyone's life has value, then your life is the most valuable of all simply because it's the only one for which you have total responsibility. You may save another person's life after a heart attack or traumatic event, but you cannot live that person's life. Your life is the only one you can live, shape, and make successful. From this perspective, your life has great value.

Just as your patients deserve the best you can give, so do you. You deserve to be honored and well cared for. You deserve a happy and successful life. But no one can care for you as well as you can. Value for yourself must come from within.

Creating and supporting a healthy self-esteem is accomplished by honoring yourself. The great Irish play-wright Oscar Wilde once said, "Fall in love with yourself and begin the romance of a lifetime." But loving yourself can be a tall order. Often, you may not feel good about yourself and your ability to be successful.

Dr. M. Scott Peck, in his best-selling book, *The Road Less Traveled,* says love is "the will to extend one's self for the purpose of nurturing one's own or another's spiritual growth." Loving yourself involves more than a general feeling; it means expressing that love and honoring your-self through uplifting thoughts and actions.

Honor Through Self-Talk

Throughout the day, we talk to ourselves through our thoughts. We carry on a constant conversation with our-selves, digesting information and offering opinions. These opinions are the foundation of our self-esteem.

To see how active your mind is, stop reading for a moment and consider how many thoughts and opinions pass through your consciousness.

The mind is a busy place. At the rapid pace of Grand Central Station, thoughts and opinions come and go. These thoughts and opinions, or self-talk, pass judgment on

More About Self-Talk

Self-talk is the term coined by psychologists for the way we instruct ourselves to relate to the world. The concept of self-talk is having an influence in such fields as psychology, neuropsychology, education, and sports psychology. Dr. Shad Helmstetter, a leading expert in self-talk, estimates that seventy-five percent of adult self-talk is negative. He points out that positive self-talk is one of the most powerful forces we have for self-transformation and taking control of our lives. You can learn more about self-talk in his popular book, *What to Say When You Talk to Yourself.*

everything in our lives. Our self-talk is a running commentary on how we regard ourselves and the world around us. In fact, it is in our thoughts or self-talk that we determine our reality.

Franklin Roosevelt once said, "The ablest man I ever met is the man you think you are." What we think about ourselves determines who and what we really are. Athletes understand this principle and use it well; they realize their performance will be directly related to their self-talk. If they go to the starting block full of doubt and

Athletes Use Self-Talk

Sprinter Florence Griffith Joyner (Flo Jo) prepared herself for the 1988 Olympics in Seoul, Korea, by using self-talk. Through mentally preparing herself, she set the world record in the women's 100 meter. She had done extremely well in the U.S. qualifying heats in Indianapolis, but when she arrived at the airport in Seoul, a luggage cart fell on her ankle bruising her Achilles tendon. For many athletes, this would have been a fatal blow. For several days before the race, Joyner could do nothing but stretch and prepare with self-talk. The night before her race, she wrote in her diary that she would run the first heat in 10.62 seconds and the final race in 10.54 seconds. When the race was called, she was ready. She exploded out of the starting blocks and ran the first heat in 10.62 seconds. She easily won the final race with a time of 10.54 seconds—exactly what she had planned.

—*From* Florence Griffith Joyner: Dazzling Olympian, *by Nathan Aaseng (Lerner Publications, Minneapolis, 1989)*

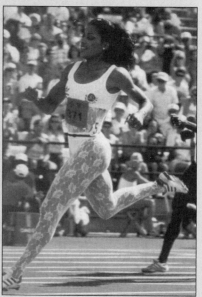

PHOTO BY CHARLES NYE/LIAISON INTERNATIONAL

negative feelings about themselves, their performance will likely suffer accordingly.

The same is true for creating success. Your attitude about yourself will influence the outcome in nearly every situation. If you develop the habit of supporting yourself with your thoughts, offering encouragement, and trusting yourself to handle whatever situation arises, you will have a positive influence on your success.

The problem is, self-talk seems hard to control. Who can control his own thoughts? Imagine going to an EMS job interview. You meet all the qualifications and fit the potential employer's needs, and the interview goes well. But several days later, the interviewer calls to tell you she's offered the job to someone more qualified than you. As you hang up the phone, your self-talk becomes wildly active. You think, "I knew I wouldn't get the job. I probably said something wrong. Was I too quiet? Maybe I should have said more about my personal goals. I'll bet it was my size. I never fit in well. Those others are just smooth talkers. I don't have what it takes. But maybe this job just wasn't for me. I'll get another chance and do better."

Thoughts race in and out of your consciousness in response to various events and situations, thoughts that may seem uncontrollable and able to hold you captive, especially if they appear to be rooted in truth. But self-talk can be managed; you can choose what you think about yourself.

Stop and think about the last time you took a written test. Even though your thoughts may have been jumbled before the test, once the test began, you chose to focus on the questions in front of you. You can manage your thoughts in other situations in the same way—by choosing which thoughts become your focus. A hundred ideas, opinions, and reactions may flash through your mind in a given situation, but you can choose which thoughts you invite to hang around.

> *"The hardest victory is the victory over self."*
> —Aristotle

In the call mentioned earlier, in which the man died from bleeding in his airway and the doctor questioned whether I had contributed to the man's death, I had a choice about my self-talk. After the doctor's comment, a storm of both positive and negative thoughts ran through my head, and for a while I doubted myself. Then I realized I had a choice: I could focus on my doubt, on the thoughts that stemmed from the fear that I was not competent, or I could focus on the fact that, regardless of what the doctor said, I had done my best. I chose the latter.

Try This:

Take a few minutes to experiment with this concept of self-talk. Regardless of what you are thinking, focus and tell yourself some positive things about yourself. If you have trouble believing your positive self-talk, tell yourself some things you wish others would say about you. Actually form words in your mind that honor you.

This is a difficult exercise. You'll notice that your mind is filled with a variety of judgmental thoughts coming from all directions. That's OK. Just keep focusing. Imagine that you are talking with a frightened patient who needs your reassurance but is hesitant to trust you. (Most of us in EMS are great at reassuring others.) Don't worry if self-deprecating or negative thoughts sneak in; simply dismiss them and form new ones. You have a choice about how you think of yourself.

Honoring yourself through self-talk is not automatic. If your self-talk tends to condemn your basic value and goodness, choosing thoughts that honor and support yourself will take practice. In taking a written test, you focus your thoughts on the questions. The questions become prompters, which help direct your thinking. In everyday life, you can focus your thoughts by developing a specific set of prompters.

Try This:

Take several 3x5 cards (we'll use a lot of them in these exercises). On each card, write a statement about yourself that will prompt positive self-talk, such as

- *I am a good person and am worthy of good things.*

- *I am competent and can handle the challenges in my life.*

- *I believe in my ability to succeed.*

- *The opinions of others are not the basis of my self-esteem.*

Carry these cards with you and read the statements at various times of the day. When you find your self-talk turning negative and judgmental of yourself, read these statements and remember that you have a choice about how you talk to yourself.

At first, monitoring your self-talk takes a great deal of concentration and can leave you feeling tired and even embarrassed. Yet how you talk to yourself is the foundation of building and maintaining a high level of self-esteem.

We will talk about many aspects of success in EMS in this book, but remember, to enjoy success in work you must first be successful in the things you say to yourself.

Honoring Yourself in Daily Actions

Several years ago, I went to the Middle East to work on an EMS development project and quickly learned about the importance of actions. Arab culture has a very different view of time and protocol in conducting business than

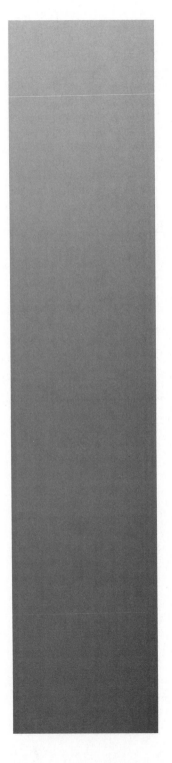

what I was accustomed to in the United States. I was in a hurry and, operating like most EMS workers, I wanted to get things moving. But Arabs like to take their time, drink some tea, and talk things over before making decisions.

Shortly after I arrived, I went to see a government official to obtain approval for a training project I was planning. I needed his blessing before anything could move forward; I saw this as an irritating formality and rushed into his office building with the necessary paper-work. As I waited outside his office for an hour, I became more and more impatient. Finally, in typically gracious Arab fashion, he greeted me at the door and invited me to come in and sit on a large, comfortable couch. He then offered me tea and began to ask about my family. I impa-tiently declined the tea, brushed off his questions, and popped open my briefcase, ready to talk business. He lis-tened patiently. When I finished and asked for his ap-proval, however, he merely sat in silence.

After a few uncomfortable minutes, I realized my mistake. But it was too late—he would approve nothing that day or for many days to come. My actions had spo-ken loudly and dishonorably. They had clearly commu-nicated that I did not honor his culture or protocol, and the result took me far from my desired outcome.

Actions communicate loudly. This is particularly true in regard to self-esteem. How you act toward yourself sends a powerful message about what you think of yourself. How you treat yourself matters. If you ignore your basic need for rest, relaxation, good nutrition, and companionship, your self-esteem will suffer.

One of the great ironies of EMS is how the workers act toward themselves. Most want to provide the best care possible for their patients, but when it comes to caring for themselves, they settle for much less. EMS workers often work long hours, go without sleep, take on extra shifts, and eat poorly. They are often inconsistent in getting

> **One of the great ironies of EMS is how the workers act toward themselves. Most want to provide the best care possible for their patients, but when it comes to caring for themselves, they settle for much less.**

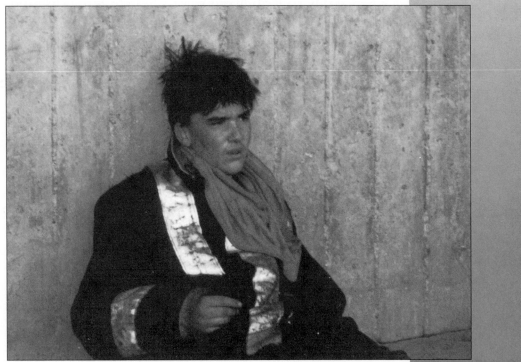

PHOTO BY JIM MALLORY/CONSULTING SYSTEMS, INC.

adequate exercise and relaxation. They frequently take on more responsibilities than they can reasonably handle. The fact is, being discouraged and negative about work goes hand-in-hand with poor self-care.

EMS workers may acknowledge the importance of self-care, but the problem is, they seem to mistake caring for others with caring for themselves. It's not uncommon, for example, to see EMS workers caring for elderly parents or alcoholic siblings. This type of caretaking, while perhaps noble, can lead them to take on extra projects, work second jobs, and be in constant motion without time or energy to care for themselves.

One of the great Greek tragedies is the story of Theseus and the Minotaur. Theseus was a young man who became the hero of his family and country by accomplishing many great, selfless, and daring feats; he was a rescuer who

> *"Nothing may be more important than being gentle with ourselves. Whether we're a professional working a sixty-hour week or a family member called upon to care for a sick relative, facing suffering continually is no small task. We learn the value of recognizing our limits, forgiving ourselves our bouts of impatience or guilt, acknowledging our own needs. We see that to have compassion for others, we must have compassion for ourselves."*
>
> —Ram Dass

roamed the roads and countryside to help people in need. But Theseus' big call came when he was sent to rescue an island from the Minotaur, a horrible monster that was half man and half bull. The Minotaur had frightened the islanders into paying an annual tribute of seven virgins, and no one was brave enough to stand up to the monster. Fearlessly, Theseus went to the island and met a beautiful maiden who instantly fell in love with him. But Theseus had a job to do, and with the woman's help, he crept up to the Minotaur while he was sleeping and killed him. It was a great victory, and Theseus returned home to a glorious celebration. But all was not well.

Through all of Theseus' rescuing, he had become so caught up in helping others that he had failed to care for himself and acknowledge what was important. All of his relationships failed, including that with his father and the beautiful maiden from the island. The remainder of his life was lonely and unhappy. So, while he had achieved great notoriety and position, Theseus failed at one of the most heroic deeds of all—caring for himself.

Many of us in EMS are like Theseus; taking care of others seems easier than caring for ourselves. We think the noble thing to do is to give and give, ultimately ignoring ourselves. Our idea of the true caregiver is one who selflessly gives to others. But as happened to Theseus, such heroic giving can leave us empty and unfulfilled. There are many EMS people who have tried to rescue and take care of everyone around them but eventually found themselves alone.

Malcolm Forbes once said, "If you don't matter to you, it's hard to matter to others." The only way we can ever really care for others is to first care for ourselves. Our value of others can only be as great as the value we have for ourselves.

Do you care for yourself? Do you demonstrate that care in action? When you practice good self-care, you're demonstrating that you believe you are valuable and worthy of good things. Self-love must be an act. How do you act toward yourself?

Try This:

Take an inventory of your actions toward yourself. Do you honor yourself in the things you do on a daily basis? Think of this as a secondary survey of your self-care. Reply to each statement with a yes or no.

1. *I make getting adequate sleep and rest a daily priority.* _____

2. *I take time to be alone with myself on a daily basis.* _____

3. *I regularly enjoy a good, hearty belly laugh.* _____

4. *I exercise or work out at least three times a week.* _____

5. *I have at least two friends who are interested in my growth.* _____

6. *I will pass up extra shifts in order to care for myself.* _____

7. *Good self-care takes precedence over caring for others.* _____

8. *My leisure and play activities are regular and satisfying.* _____

9. *Good nutrition and a balanced diet are daily habits.* _____

10. *I make working toward my dreams a daily activity.* _____

Look over your answers and take time to reflect on the things you would like to change about the way you care for yourself.

When you practice good self-care, you're demonstrating that you believe you are valuable and worthy of good things.

You may try to rationalize poor self-care by saying: "I just don't have time for myself. I have bills to pay, a fam-

"When experiencing difficulty in discerning your own needs, it may be helpful to begin by observing what you provide for others. Often we give to other people what we unconsciously know we need ourselves."

—Carmen Renee Berry

ily to care for, and a career to build." During my early years in EMS, I failed miserably in caring for myself. It seemed noble and admirable to work hard and go without food, sleep, and exercise. I had the expenses of a new family and believed I could ignore my own physical and emotional needs while caring for everyone else.

By my fifth year in EMS, I had a lingering stomach ulcer and a painful low-back injury. I was depressed about my work and was tired all the time. Like most medical people, I focused on the symptoms. I took medication for the ulcer, went to physical therapy for the back, and tried to ignore the depression. But none of it worked; as soon as I stopped the treatment, the symptoms returned.

For a time, I was convinced I would have to leave EMS to feel better—a common assumption among EMS workers who don't practice good self-care. But finally, through the counsel of some good friends and a determination to have a better life, I began to make self-care a priority. I started by eating healthy foods every day and exercising at least four times a week.

I couldn't believe the difference. By simply making changes in diet and committing to exercise, I found new energy. As my physical condition improved, so did my health. My mental and emotional condition improved as well.

In the long run, taking the time to care for yourself will make you much more productive and successful. At first it may seem laborious and extremely selfish, but as time goes on and you develop the habit of self-care, you will notice a gradual boost in your self-esteem. As you begin to like yourself more, you will feel more in touch with the things you really want and will experience a noticeable increase in energy.

Learning to honor yourself through daily actions can be difficult; changing old habits is not easy. So begin slowly. Pick three ways to practice caring for yourself, and commit to them for three weeks. At the end of three weeks, evaluate the effects.

A good way to start is by taking a daily "time-out." Set aside a short period of time each day to get away from all your responsibilities and the many things you "should" be doing. Use this time just to think, order your day, read, or write in a journal. Establish a specific time each day, and remember, stick with it for three weeks. The rewards will be many. EMS workers who practice daily time-outs find themselves in closer touch with what they need.

Another way to start caring for yourself is to limit the hours you work each week. In EMS, there is always a temptation to pick up extra shifts, teach another class, or even

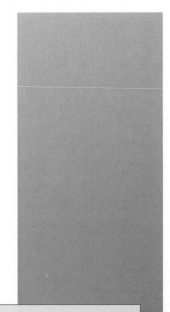

The Mind-Body Connection

Regular exercise and low cholesterol and weight levels are not the only determinants of good health, according to Ruth Stricker, a nationally recognized fitness and wellness authority. Stricker offers five suggestions for developing a balanced approach to taking care of yourself.

1. Think positive. "Show a sense of humor. Laugh. Use moderation and common sense. Respect life on this planet."
2. Relax. "Some people get so uptight with their workouts that they negate any health benefits."
3. Stay fit. "I don't mean beating up your body. I don't mean working out six days a week. I'm talking about staying in fighting shape. Keep your body in shape for surgery, to fight disease, and most certainly to decrease the effects of stress or aging. That means having vitality in the body."
4. Enrich your mind. "How? Through mental exercises. Through reading and thinking with friends—and through the arts."
5. Save the world. "In other words, altruism. I'm convinced that we can get a helper's high. That's as important as nutrition or exercise. We have to get outside ourselves; it is a part of wellness."

—*From* Minnesota Monthly, *January 1994, p. 54*

work a second job. But overworking can deprive you of rest, relaxation, and perspective. In contrast, limiting your work can have dramatic results. Instead of thinking only about financial needs and how to make more money, limit your work and begin to work smarter. You will gain a more realistic focus on what you really want from your career and life. You will feel better about yourself and improve your self-esteem. By not overworking, priorities will become clear, and the energy for dreaming will return. Limiting how much you work is a powerful way to honor yourself.

Another area of self-care that will bring rapid results is regular exercise. A good physical workout has many positive effects: It improves how you feel physically, increases energy and alertness, builds self-confidence, and seems to have a noticeable impact on depression.

Regular exercise is essential in EMS work. It combats the lethargic feeling of shift work and takes the irritating edge off the frustration that comes from waiting for the unknown. Regular exercise is also critical to a good self-concept. Choose an exercise or sport that you enjoy, and start slowly.

Yet another area of self-care is play. Someone once said, "We don't stop playing because we grow old; we grow old because we stop playing." The happiest EMS workers are the ones who continually keep a spirit of playfulness and laughter in their lives and work. Do you allow yourself to play? Do you regularly do something just for the fun and playfulness of it?

I once worked for a service where Frisbees and water balloons (made from latex gloves) were standard equipment on each rig. Between the difficult calls, people played. During downtime, we had elaborate Frisbee games and played practical jokes on other crews.

Because there is such a sober side to EMS work, play is essential. Singing, telling jokes, drawing pictures, tossing a Frisbee, or making something with your hands can all kindle the sheer joy of being alive.

Along with play comes humor. Have you ever noticed how much better you feel after you have a good, deep belly laugh? Stop and think about the laugh itself. You throw back your head, your mouth opens wide, and you let loose with a primitive sound that goes beyond any language. When you laugh, something happens in your body, mind, and spirit that is refreshing and honors your very existence. Make it a point to have one of those deep, shaking belly laughs every day. It's an easy goal, and such a habit is a powerful action toward honoring yourself.

There are countless ways you can practice good self-care. (Additional resources for developing good self-care are listed at the end of this chapter.) Regardless of the self-care you practice, assess it often by considering how you feel about yourself. If you are feeling down and discouraged and are critical of yourself and everyone else, stop and check how you're treating yourself.

Caring for yourself is an act of love. It also has a powerful impact on your success, reinforcing that you are important and are endowed with everything you need to succeed in EMS and life.

The basics of self-talk and honoring yourself will be as critical to your success as the basic skills of EMS. On an emergency call, when everything goes wrong and you're unsure of what to do, you can always turn to the ABCs of basic life support. Similarly, as your career leads you down many paths and through many difficult situations, returning to the basics will help you rediscover the focus you need.

Summary

✔ Success in EMS begins with YOU and your belief in yourself.

> When you laugh, something happens in your body, mind, and spirit that is refreshing and honors your very existence.

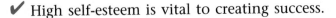

✔ High self-esteem is vital to creating success.

✔ EMS is not a cure for low self-esteem.

✔ The nature of EMS work can promote self-doubt.

✔ High self-esteem is built from the inside out through honoring yourself.

✔ Honor yourself through positive self-talk.

✔ Honor yourself in your daily actions toward yourself.

Suggested Reading

Honoring the Self, by Nathaniel Branden (Bantam Books, New York, 1983). A practical guide to honoring yourself from the inside out with supporting material on the importance of self-esteem.

The Power of Self-Esteem, by Nathaniel Branden (Health Communications, Inc., Deerfield Beach, Florida, 1992). This book provides a comprehensive look at self-esteem and how it affects us—especially in the area of our achievements.

The Road Less Traveled, by M. Scott Peck, M.D. (Simon and Schuster, New York, 1978). This best-selling classic is a powerful guide to getting in touch with yourself and what you really want. M. Scott Peck is a psychiatrist without the medical lingo. Using what he's learned in his practice, he demonstrates the essentials of a mentally and spiritually healthy life.

Smart Exercise, by Covert Bailey (Houghton Mifflin Company, New York, 1994). Of all the material available on nutrition, exercise, and staying in shape, it's difficult to find something practical and truly useful. Covert Bailey, from the popular PBS series entitled *Covert Bailey's Fit or Fat*, knows what's important when it comes to staying in shape. If you are serious about staying fit but sick of the fads, this book is the answer. This is the best buy for both fitness and nutritional help.

The Way of the Peaceful Warrior, by Dan Millman (H. J. Kramer, Inc., Tiburon, California, 1980). Dan Millman is an athlete and a great storyteller. He teaches how you can reclaim control of your life and truly begin to honor yourself in the way you live.

What to Say When You Talk to Yourself, by Shad Helmstetter (Pocket Books, New York, 1982). Shad Helmstetter is much more than a motivational writer. He has examined how to realize your potential for success from the practical and applicable perspective of self-talk. The book teaches just what the title suggests.

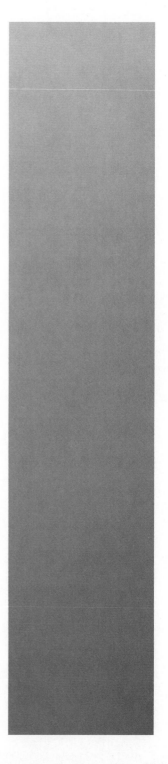

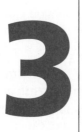

3 Clarifying Your Purpose

Your work is to discover your work and then, with all your heart, give yourself to it.

—The Buddha

It was a routine flight from Denver to Chicago when, suddenly, one of the DC-10's engines exploded. The force of the explosion blasted shrapnel into the plane's steering and control systems, and Captain Al Haynes found himself piloting a plane that would not respond to the controls. There was no way to steer or slow the plane, and United Airlines Flight 242 appeared to be doomed.

Despite the hopelessness of the situation, Haynes did not give up. Using all of his experience, knowledge, and resources, he focused on the clear and vital purpose of getting his 292 passengers safely to the ground. Nothing else mattered.

Calmly, Haynes radioed his problem. None of the engineers at the emergency flight service center were able to help him find a solution, so it was agreed that he should head for the Sioux City, Iowa, airport and attempt a landing. With co-pilot Bill Records and flight engineer Dudley Devorak, Haynes devised a plan to steer the jet by vary-

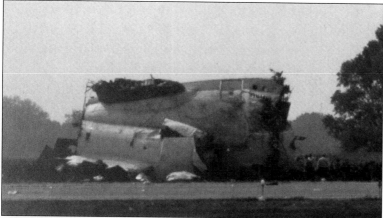

PHOTOS BY MICHAEL SPRINGER/LIAISON INTERNATIONAL

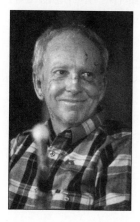

Al Haynes, captain of United Flight 242, speaks at a press conference days after the crash at Sioux City, Iowa. Thanks to Haynes' skill, 184 people survived the disaster.

ing the thrust of the two remaining engines. It was a crude attempt to control the jet, but somehow Haynes made it work well enough to keep the craft in the air.

When the Sioux City tower reported that the runways had been cleared for a landing, Haynes casually betrayed the desperate nature of his situation by replying, "You want to be particular and make it a runway, huh? I'm just aiming for Iowa."

Haynes' purpose enabled him to do the impossible, and he carefully hobbled the crippled plane toward the Sioux City airport. He knew he would only have one try at the landing, as did the emergency crews, which waited on the ground, expecting the worst. But with unbelievable accuracy, the plane came down toward the runway for a crash landing.

There was no way to slow the plane, and as it hit the ground it bounced, cartwheeled, and exploded into flames.

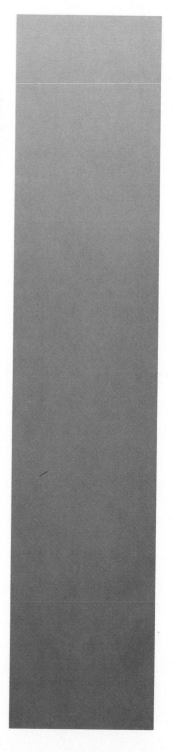

"The secret of success is constancy to purpose."

—Benjamin Disraeli

"A goal is something tangible; a purpose is a direction. A goal can be achieved; a purpose is fulfilled in each moment."

—John-Roger and Peter McWilliams

Having a clear and vital purpose produces amazing results.

A total of 112 people died, but amazingly, because of Haynes' heroic efforts, 184 people survived.

Later, in more than forty computer-simulated attempts, not one pilot could duplicate Haynes' maneuvers.

As Captain Haynes demonstrated, having a clear and vital purpose produces amazing results. This principle is seen every day in EMS work. A rescuer may be tired and unmotivated and dreaming of paradise, but when a call for help comes, he suddenly finds purpose and can rise to whatever the situation demands. When we have a reason, we find a way.

The same is true when considering the big picture of EMS. When you clarify your purpose for being in this work, you get in touch with the experience you really want. Purpose focuses you on the particular aspects of the work that are interesting and rewarding to you. More than just becoming the best in EMS, personal success means finding and creating what you as an individual want from this work. What issues are important to you? What aspects of this work ignite your life? If you could custom-design your EMS experience, what would it look like?

What Is Purpose?

Purpose is life's motivation; it is the reason for being—or, for that matter, doing. Purpose is what gets us up in the morning. Having a purpose is what empowers us and ultimately leads to satisfaction and fulfillment in our lives and work.

In his book *The Power of Purpose,* Richard Leider writes: "Having purpose in our lives means that something (an aim, a goal, an interest, a person, an idea) attracts us enough to move us to action on its behalf and is important enough so that focusing on it orders our activities and provides our lives with a sense of meaning. Purpose helps me understand what is relevant to my life, what it is I live for, who I am, and what I am about in actual day-to-day living. My world makes some sense to me."

On the surface, our reasons for doing the things we do may seem obvious. If asked why you want to work in EMS, you might respond, "I want work that is exciting and helpful to others." But there's more to your purpose. What do you consider exciting work? Why do you want to help others? Why EMS and not engineering, business, international diplomacy, or even police work or firefighting? How does EMS fit with your personal values? What is it about this work that you find satisfying and rewarding? These questions will take you beyond the surface to where your real motivation or purpose lies.

Purpose is a combination of who you are and your deepest desires and core values. Purpose rests at the very center of who you are as a person. The problem is, we rarely take the time to understand what really motivates us, which leaves us with a cloudy understanding of how to create success.

The Benefits of Clarifying Purpose

When people get a grasp on the "why" of their work, the puzzle pieces of success begin to fit together. Let's consider why a clear sense of purpose is so important.

Having Purpose Is Essential to Survival

A surgeon with a University of Minnesota organ transplant team said he was convinced a person's attitude is the greatest predictor of transplant survival. "My patients who have a purpose to live find the energy and will to fight," he said. "Regardless of the medical care, having a reason to live is critical to survival."

People who survive great adversity talk about the importance of purpose. During his eight long years of captivity as a hostage in Lebanon, journalist Terry Anderson said the hope of seeing his wife and child kept him

> *"The concept of purpose is not an end point but a process. It is not a description of the last days of your life, but of its continuing saga from this moment on, into a future as you would have it be if you could determine it. And you can!"*
>
> —Richard J. Leider

alive. He had a purpose. The same is true in EMS work—while it should not be a long, awful ordeal, EMS is difficult work, and having a purpose is critical to long-term survival.

Unfortunately, EMS people often leave the field in the midst of difficulties, whether they are personal problems, trouble with management, or even a string of bad calls. They don't allow their sense of purpose to see them through. If there is no clear purpose, survival in anything seems pointless. In contrast, when you know why you are doing something, you are much more likely to endure.

Clarifying Purpose Links Dreams With Reality

We all have dreams, and we often express our dreams by saying, "If I had a million dollars, I would . . . " or "If I could do anything in the world I wanted, I would. . . ." Perhaps we call them dreams because they seem like childish fantasies—unreal and completely out of touch with our everyday lives. But dreams are more than just wishful thinking. Everything created begins with a dream, including your success in EMS. Your dreams have a lot to say about what you want from life and what form your success will take. When you clarify purpose, you begin building a bridge between dreams and reality. Dreams are the travel brochures to your success.

One of the first paramedics in the Los Angeles area in the late 1960s was a man named John Bateman. John enjoyed EMS work and was good at it, but he also had a desire to travel the world. At first, the reality of EMS and his dream to travel seemed incompatible; John was not wealthy and did not want to give up his hard-earned career in EMS. But in clarifying his purpose, he acknowledged his dream. Instead of accepting that EMS and world travel were incompatible, he began to bridge the gap between his dream and reality.

I recently met up with John in Cairo, Egypt, in the

If there is no clear purpose, survival in anything seems pointless.

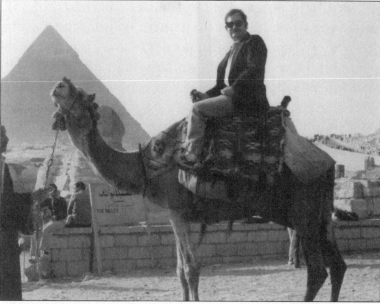

PHOTO COURTESY OF JOHN BATEMAN

John Bateman has made his dream of world travel compatible with a career in EMS.

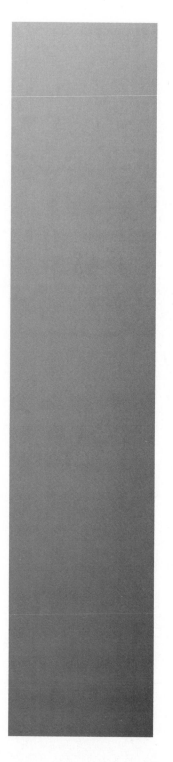

middle of yet another trip around the world. For more than twenty years, he has worked in EMS-related jobs all over the world and has traveled to countless countries. He has enjoyed one of the most diverse experiences possible and yet has maintained his connections to EMS. John's experience has not been the result of easy breaks or chance, but of a clear purpose focused in the direction of his dreams.

A Clear Purpose Leads, Directs, and Focuses Energy

Because EMS is a relatively new career field, the "career path" is not well-defined. What will you do after five years as a street paramedic? Not knowing exactly where to go with an EMS career is a frustrating journey into uncharted waters. While part of the reason for this frustration may be the evolving nature of EMS, a bigger part may be a failure to clarify what you really want.

In the beginning, EMS promises to be exciting and rewarding work, but the excitement will not last forever. "I just don't know what to do next," is a common complaint among veteran EMS workers. But purpose is necessary for direction. In a 1988 *Reader's Digest* article titled "Street Smart Secrets for Success," David Mahoney writes: "Without a personal philosophy, a strong perception of who you are and what you stand for, you get buffeted around by every person, message, idea, and event that comes down the pike. You'll find yourself running off in all directions at once."

A clear sense of purpose leads, directs, and tells you where to focus your energy. Imagine going to a scene in which a man has been shot in the face and chest with a shotgun. He has airway problems and a possible pneumothorax. The scene is noisy and chaotic: The man's wife is screaming, a dog is barking, and an entire army of police officers is shouting about the need to preserve the crime scene for evidence. In addition, it's the end of a long shift, and you are tired and want to go home.

In the midst of all this chaos, you focus on what needs to be done. You kneel beside the man and quickly evaluate his ABCs. You assess the airway and begin to ventilate. Your purpose is clear: You want to keep the man's brain well-oxygenated until you reach the ED. As you work, you have all the energy you need. Almost effortlessly, you help boost the patient onto the backboard. One of the police officers wants you to do something about the man's superficial bleeding, but your purpose directs you to continue to manage the airway. On other calls you might stop to reassure the wife, but the greater mission of keeping the patient alive directs you to move with him. Hardly thinking, you have taken charge of the entire scene, directing people to move things out of the way and help carry the backboard. Because your purpose is crystal clear, you know exactly what to do.

A clear sense of purpose leads, directs, and tells you where to focus your energy.

In your career and life, a clear purpose has the same effect. Knowing why you do something, as well as what you want and how it relates to your values, will lead, direct, and focus your energies.

Clarifying Purpose Leads to Meaning and Reward

Finally, clarifying purpose gives meaning to our lives. Most of us want lives that are more than a 70-year struggle to exist, and we want our work to be more than just a means of earning money. Beyond the rather temporary rewards of excitement and adventure, *meaning* is the real reward in EMS. Few of us get rich in this work; we do it because we expect it to be meaningful. But without a clear sense of purpose, there is no meaning, and consequently, no reward.

One paramedic who had decided to quit EMS said, "When I came to EMS, I thought it would be great work, but it's turned out to be a lot different than I imagined. The pay isn't great, there's no future, and besides, management is always hassling us about stuff that doesn't matter. It just doesn't pay."

When asked what attracted him to the business in the first place, he replied, "I guess I'm like everyone else. I was an action junkie and a siren head. I wanted good calls and lots of trauma. I thought it was cool to help people, and for a while it was. It felt great to work an arrest and get someone back. But now I guess I've seen all the action and excitement I want. Most of the time, I'm not sure my skills make much difference in the patient's outcome. I've discovered that no one really cares if I do a good job or not. I take a lot of time putting on a splint, and when I get to the ED, a doctor rips it off. No one seems to respect what I do, so why should I? Besides that, after a while, you realize you're not unique. There are a bunch of people breaking down the door to take my job, and for all I know, management would be as happy with them as with me."

> *"As a medic in Vietnam, I naturally slipped into EMS work, thinking it was a logical career choice after the Army—nothing more. But now, looking back over 20 years, I can see there was a lot more to my becoming a medic than just making a practical career choice. There was something deep inside of me that wanted to help people, be needed, and have a sense of satisfaction about my work. I'm not sure I can spell it out, but I can sure see it now as I look back."*
>
> —A veteran paramedic

"I can't even tell you what color the house was or how big it was. There were two kids who weren't breathing—that's all I needed to know. We just went to work on those kids. I don't even think I looked up at the fire after that."

—An EMT firefighter

Granted, this paramedic said many important things about the state of some EMS operations, but more important, he revealed something about his own purpose. His purpose had changed and become unclear to him. Once he acknowledged his insatiable desire for excitement and realized that helping people is not always glorious or exciting, his purpose became clouded. Without a clear sense of purpose, his work had no meaning. It became frustrating and laborious and ceased to be rewarding.

During World War II, the people of London, England, endured almost constant bombing by German aircraft. Air raid sirens sounded daily, and people would run for underground bomb shelters. Sometimes they would crowd together for days at a time in conditions that were crude and confining. They lived in fear and faced destruction and even death. Life was unpredictable. Yet years later, many of the people who lived through that period reported that the Battle for Britain was the most meaningful and rewarding time of their lives. Why?

During that dark period of history, daily life for Londoners had a powerful purpose. They were literally fighting for their lives and freedom. Where there is purpose, meaning and reward will follow.

Even in life's more mundane, albeit aggravating, situations, you will find that having a clear purpose can help you cope. Recently, my wife came home with a dangerous brake problem on her car. It was too late to get the car into the shop that day, and she needed the car the next morning. I do not like working on cars. I swear a lot and wind up with skinned knuckles and a poor attitude. However, I've repaired enough cars to know how to fix a few things.

So I pulled on some old clothes and crawled around under her car for three hours. It wasn't easy work. In fact, it was not at all fun. I swore a lot, bloodied my knuckles, and even broke a few tools. But the work was meaningful, and when I was done, I had a satisfying sense of reward. I had not suddenly fallen in love with car repair, but I was convinced of my purpose. I wanted my wife to have a safe car to drive the next morning. Having a clear purpose made a frustrating job meaningful and rewarding.

Personal Leadership

Throughout our lives, we have crisis experiences that will clarify purpose for us, as happened with Captain Haynes, Terry Anderson, and the failing brakes. Often a death, a sudden tragic event, or even a divorce or a job loss can suddenly make our purpose in life crystal clear. In fact, in the midst of a crisis, we let go of petty concerns, conflicts, and our desire for fame and fortune. In a crisis, every moment becomes precious, and we can clearly see what's important.

Many EMS workers live their lives waiting for something to happen. They wait for the next call, the right job, or a big break. But why wait for a crisis? You can willfully begin to clarify your purpose by taking a leadership role in your life. Clarifying purpose is an act of per-

---

Personal Leadership Versus Management

- **Personal Leadership**
  Concerned with doing the right thing.
  What is my purpose?
  What should I do?
  Where am I going?

- **Personal Management**
  Concerned with doing things right.
  What are my specific goals?
  How should I do it?
  How should I get there?

You can willfully begin to clarify your purpose by taking a leadership role in your life.

sonal leadership. It's about leading your EMS career instead of just managing it.

Leadership and management may seem similar, but they are two very different concepts. Imagine a group of people hiking through the mountains. The managers in the group will be concerned about how the hike is going. Are people keeping up? Is there enough water? The managers will organize the rest periods and make sure feet don't become blistered. They will assign people to the different tasks of setting up camp. Managers are concerned about getting things done right.

The leaders have a very different role. They are concerned about where the group is going. They have a dream and a vision about the destination. Occasionally, they leave the group to check out the trail or climb up high hills to look ahead. They keep an eye on the weather and decide which fork in the road to take. Often, they run back to the hikers and managers to remind them of where they're going and how beautiful it will be when they arrive. They share their dreams of the destination and remain focused on the big picture. Leaders are concerned about where they are going, not just how they will get there.

Leadership in your own life and work is the same way. Just as hikers need leadership, your work in EMS needs your leadership. And the best way to begin leading is by clarifying your purpose.

The Process of Clarifying Purpose

You may shrug off the idea of clarifying your purpose by saying, "I know why I'm in EMS and what I want from this work—it's all clear to me." But what may seem obvious may be masking something deeper.

A number of years ago, I went on a call for a young motorcyclist who had been struck by a pickup truck. The truck's bumper had smashed into the side of the motorcycle, crushing the young man's leg and sending him fly-

Leaders are concerned about where they are going, not just how they will get there.

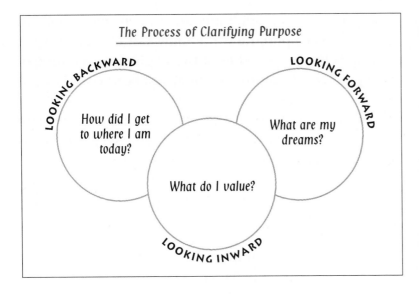

The Process of Clarifying Purpose

LOOKING BACKWARD

LOOKING FORWARD

How did I get to where I am today?

What are my dreams?

What do I value?

LOOKING INWARD

ing into a ditch. He was conscious and screaming from the pain of his leg injury when my partner and I arrived. He had an open fracture of the femur with significant bleeding, and the lower leg was pulverized. The bones were shattered into more than thirty pieces. As I cut off the man's boot, his leg felt like Jell-O. It was one of the worst leg injuries I'd ever seen. My partner and I stabilized and splinted the leg with PASG and started for the hospital.

On the way to the hospital, the man suddenly began to pale. I checked the bleeding from the upper leg and was confident I had it controlled, but the man's condition seemed to worsen. His eyes grew wide, and he looked terrified. I knew something was seriously wrong but couldn't figure it out until he began to struggle with his breathing. Then it hit me. In my foolish focus on the leg, I had missed a pneumothorax. I had failed to complete a thorough secondary survey.

Clarifying your purpose is a lot like conducting a secondary survey—many people are distracted by what appears to be obvious. The secondary survey is a process that begins at the head and works to the toes; this thorough

"Change and growth take place when a person has risked himself and dares to become involved with his own life."

—Herbert Otto

Looking backward is about looking at your life and reflecting on how you have come to be where you are today.

process ensures you don't miss the less obvious problems. Clarifying your purpose is the same sort of process. Each part must be completed for a thorough understanding of your purpose—a purpose that may not be as visible as you think.

For the next part of this chapter, find a quiet place where you won't be disturbed. Clarifying your purpose is a very personal and intense process that deserves your full attention. The process includes three looks: a look backward, a look forward, and a look inward.

Looking Backward

One of the most important components of a patient survey is gathering the patient's medical history and the history of the present event. Similarly, in clarifying purpose, your personal history contains important data. While you may underestimate the value of your history, it is a unique story which, when honored, will reveal wonderful clues about what motivates you, what draws you to this work and, ultimately, what rewards you are seeking. Looking backward is about looking at your life and reflecting on how you have come to be where you are today.

Try This:

Looking Backward Worksheet

Take some time to reflect on what brought you to EMS. The following questions will guide you through examining your personal history. Think carefully about each of the questions and then write down your answers. The process of writing will help you be precise.

　　1. Why are you interested in EMS? What drew you to this work? Mention some of the important events in your life that led you to pursue work in EMS.

　　———————————————————

　　———————————————————

2. What life experiences have been most satisfying and rewarding?

_____

_____

3. What work experiences have you found to be satisfying and rewarding?

_____

_____

4. What work experiences have you found to be the most frustrating?

_____

_____

5. What work experiences have brought you the most happiness? Describe the situation, events, or circumstances.

_____

_____

6. When you first considered working in EMS, what sort of activities and experiences did you imagine finding?

_____

_____

7. Who have your heroes been throughout your life? How were they heroic?

_____

_____

8. Draw a time line that stretches from your high school graduation to today. Plot all of your significant life events, including moments at which you felt the most fulfilled and those points of important growth and change.

Once you finish answering these questions, read what

you've written and take a few minutes to consider what your history tells you about your purpose in EMS.

Looking Forward

EMS is moment-to-moment work. The day's activities are difficult to predict; no one knows when, where, or what the next call will be. Even with the computer forecasting of system status management, no one can predict calls accurately. Therefore, due to the nature of EMS, planning ahead has limitations. All you know for sure is that emergencies will happen and EMS workers will respond.

Because of the reactionary nature of EMS, forward thinking and planning are not rewarded, and many EMS workers are vague about what they want their futures to entail. Although this wait-and-see attitude must prevail in daily EMS work, it need not prevail in long-term career planning.

What do you want from your EMS work? You may get caught up in the business of managing daily life and lose sight of the future, but your concept of the future will have a huge impact on how you live each day. What is your vision of the future? What you see is part of your purpose.

A number of years ago, I dreamed of practicing EMS in an international setting. I imagined not only applying my skills in a setting where they were really needed, but I also wanted to see how EMS was practiced around the world. At first it was only a dream, as I had no idea of how to make it come true or whether it was even possible. In fact, I knew no one in international EMS. But I continued to allow myself to think about international work, and slowly that led to action. It was not easy, but after some careful planning, my dream became a reality. I eventually worked on EMS projects in the Middle East and Central America.

Your dreams represent your deepest desires and can lead you beyond the things you think you *should* do to the things you really *want* to do. Dreams form the mind's vision of how it will create the future.

Try This:

Looking Forward Worksheet

Now that you've reviewed your personal history, go to the next step and consider the future. Don't hurry through this part. Complete the following questions as truthfully as possible, and take your time. Give yourself permission to look as far ahead and as far afield as your dreams will allow. As before, be sure to write answers to each of the questions.

1. *What do you want to accomplish in relation to EMS in the immediate future? What are your immediate aspirations?*

   _____

   _____

2. *Regardless of your current situation, allow yourself to dream for a few moments. What are your dreams in relation to your EMS work?*

   _____

   _____

3. *Go beyond your current concerns for a job. If you could do anything you wanted, what would it be? (There's no need to be practical—have fun.)*

   _____

   _____

4. *Imagine being retired and going for a walk one day. As you head down the street, you hear an approaching siren, and you stop and watch a flashy new ambulance race by. The ambulance causes you to reflect on your EMS experiences. How do you want to remember your work in EMS? What do you want to be able to say*

Dreams form the mind's vision of how it will create the future.

about it? Years from now, what do you hope to tell a grandson or granddaughter about your EMS experience?

_____

_____

5. *Imagine being given an award in the future for life-time accomplishments in EMS. What sort of things would that award include? No matter how simple or grand, write down the accomplishments for which you want recognition.*

_____

_____

6. *Apart from EMS, what are your dreams? Apart from rescue work, what do you want to do with your life?*

_____

_____

7. *Draw a timeline of your future. Make a line, and at the far left write your current age. Then mark the line in five-year increments up to age 75. Now fill in things you would like to do or accomplish at various ages. Have fun! You are beginning to lead your life.*

Now that you've completed your look ahead, go back over your answers and reflect on what they tell you about your purpose in EMS. How does EMS fit into your dreams? What sort of future are you allowing yourself to have?

> **Your values are at the core of what truly brings meaning and satisfaction.**

Looking Inward

A clarification of your purpose would be meaningless without looking inward to your values. Values reflect those things you believe and hold dear. Values are the personal principles that guide your life. No matter what your history or your dreams, your values are at the core of what truly brings meaning and satisfaction. Values have a profound effect on how you live your life. In examining your values, the unique part of you shows through.

The idea for the following exercise comes from Stephen Covey's book about personal leadership called, *The Seven Habits of Highly Effective People*. This exercise has been proven to have a powerful effect on anyone who takes the time to complete it.

Try This:

Looking Inward Worksheet

Take your time with this exercise. It may be difficult to complete, but stick with it. It is about your life and what is most important to you. After reflecting, don't neglect to write down your answers. Putting your reflections on paper will make them more real to your subconscious mind.

Imagine you are attending a funeral and that the funeral is yours. The setting is quiet, and many of your friends and family have gathered to pay their last respects. They are sad, but they also want to remember you as you really lived. As the service begins, several people rise to speak amid the bouquets of flowers. What will they say about you? How will they say you lived your life? What will they say about your work, the way you spent your time or the way you treated other people? What characteristics will they describe? What words—honest, loyal, kind, joyful, caring, fun, inspirational—will they use to describe you? What impact will you have had on their lives?

1. Take some time and write a eulogy for yourself. (Your name) was a person who. . . .

2. Now look at your eulogy. What do you want to be remembered for? What are your values? At the core of who you are, what is most important to you? Make a list of your values.

Example: 1. To care about others
2. To be happy and content
3. To be a good person

Writing Your Mission Statement for EMS

Having completed the look forward, backward, and inward, you now have the research needed to begin clarifying your purpose in EMS and writing a personal mission statement. Your mission statement is simply a written declaration of your purpose in EMS as you see it right now. A mission statement is not carved in stone. It should, and will, change. Remember, this process of looking backward, forward, and inward is not something you do once. It should be repeated many times as you reach different stages in your EMS experience.

Constructing your personal mission statement need not be done in one sitting. In fact, your mission statement may go through a number of revisions, but it is important to actually start writing.

To begin, review the three worksheets and spend some time reflecting on what you wrote. Make some notes or highlight important points, and then simply begin writing a paragraph that begins with this phrase: *My personal mission in EMS is to. . . .*

There is no right or wrong way to do this. Just make sure you include what is relevant from your history, your dreams, and your values. You can make a list, number points, or write sentences. I've included some other EMS workers' mission statements to help you get started.

My personal mission in EMS is to work in a setting that is not boring and that allows me to work with people and be respected. I will always do the best for my patients and treat the people around me with compassion and respect. Some of the things I wish to accomplish in this field are

- *To work in a busy, respected ALS service with many challenging calls*

- *To explore my interest in teaching*
- *To use my interest in mechanical things for the betterment of the field*
- *To make enough money to live comfortably and have a family*
- *To continue to explore other occupations*

I want to treat others fairly, always give my best to the people I care for, and be trusted and respected by the people I work for.

My personal mission in EMS is to pursue my love of rescue work. It is my intention to learn as much as I can about emergency work and then apply my knowledge in leading others. I want to be known as a person who is fair, loyal, and hardworking. I want my work in EMS to be challenging and growth-oriented. I will seek opportunities in which I can explore management and leadership roles.

> *"Your imagination is your preview of life's coming attractions."*
>
> —Albert Einstein

As you begin to write your mission statement, don't be discouraged if you find yourself resisting the process. Discomfort is always associated with growth, and clarifying your purpose is truly a growing experience. Your first draft will not be perfect, but give yourself permission to finish it. Once a draft is completed, put it aside, but only for a day. Then pick it up the next day and write another draft. Remember, this mission statement is for you. Make it fit your style. Just make certain it truly reflects your history, your dreams, and your values.

Applying Your Purpose

Once you're satisfied with your mission statement,

copy it onto a 3x5 card or something that is convenient to carry with you. Review your mission statement at least once a day, and reflect on the choices and decisions you will make that day. As you internalize your mission statement, some amazing things will start to happen. You will begin to make decisions based not on what is easiest, but on what you really want. You will begin to see your values directing your responses and reactions. Over time, you will start to recognize short- and long-term goals, and you will begin to have the energy to make them into realities.

Many years ago, when I wrote my first mission statement, I remember being worried I wouldn't live up to my own expectations. The experience of putting my mission in writing was difficult and somewhat disconcerting. I even felt a little guilty for spending so much time on myself. But in working through the process, I made a number of discoveries.

Over the years, my mission in EMS has changed significantly. Like most newcomers to the field, in the beginning I was looking for an endless stream of excitement. But excitement is an interesting desire—it's often insatiable and frequently not found when directly pursued. With time, my mission has become more reflective and inclusive of the person I am and want to be. Currently, my mission for my EMS work is as follows:

> *My mission in EMS is to use the emergency setting to make a difference—no matter how small—in my world. I will strive to use my gifts and talents to better the people I'm called on to help, as well as my co-workers and myself. I will view each call as an opportunity, and I will strive to live each shift as if it were my last. I will balance my EMS experience with other outside activities and experiences that honor myself, my dreams, and my family. I will strive to*

make a positive contribution to the paramedic profession and to make the job better for those who come after me. I will continue to build community and respect among the people I work with. I will seek ways in which I can help the larger world recognize the contribution and dedication of EMS workers. I will work with pride and never minimize my work or allow myself to disrespect my choice of work regardless of the response of others.

Henry David Thoreau wrote, "If a man advances confidently in the direction of his dreams to live the life he has imagined, he will meet with a success unexpected in common hours." Creating success is stimulating. Instead of feeling helpless and at the mercy of life's ups and downs, you can begin to lead your life and career in a direction that will truly be successful.

> *"What lies behind us and what lies before us are tiny matters compared to what lies within us."*
>
> —Oliver Wendell Holmes

Summary

✔ Creating success in EMS demands having a clear sense of purpose.

✔ Purpose is a combination of your deepest desires and core values.

✔ Purpose is essential to survival, to connecting with dreams, to direction, to finding meaning.

✔ Clarifying purpose is an act of personal leadership.

✔ Purpose in EMS work is not created, it's discovered.

✔ Purpose is clarified by looking backward, forward, and inward.

✔ A personal mission statement is the way to capture your purpose.

Suggested Reading

Do What You Love and the Money Will Follow, by Marsha Sinetar (Paulist Press, Mahwah, New Jersey, 1987). This book is not the typical "get rich quick" guide. Marsha Sinetar is a psychologist who makes a great argument for doing what you really want. She shows how people who follow their dream livelihood end up learning how to support themselves—an idea greatly needed in EMS work.

Illusions, by Richard Bach (Dell Publishing, New York, 1977). This is a story about a man who confronts his purpose in life. It is a great read and a wonderful way to begin looking at your life and work from a totally new perspective.

The Path of the Everyday Hero, by Lorna Catford and Michael Ray (Tarcher Books, Los Angeles, 1991). This is an excellent workbook to help you discover your purpose. It uses fairy tales and myths to take you through a process of clarifying your purpose and discovering what you really want.

The Power of Purpose, by Richard Leider (Ballantine Books, New York, 1985). This book is a short read but extremely valuable in understanding the importance of purpose and how to discover it.

Wishcraft: How to Get What You Really Want, by Barbara Sher (Ballantine Books, New York, 1983). Barbara Sher is a single mother who started with nothing and yet began to fulfill her own wishes for life. Her book is a fun guide to mapping your own path and fulfilling your dreams. Many people today are living their dreams because of this book.

4 The Successful Job Campaign

The major difference between successful and unsuccessful job hunters is the way they go about their job hunt—and not some factor "out there," such as a tight labor market.

—Richard Nelson Bolles

In the early morning hours of December 7, 1941, 360 Japanese planes descended on the Hawaiian Islands in a devastating surprise attack. In less than an hour, the U.S. Pacific fleet was nearly destroyed. Scores of ships had been sunk or damaged, and 3,435 people were dead or injured. As news of the attack spread, Americans became incensed by the brutality of it. They wanted immediate revenge. President Roosevelt declared war on Japan, but a swift victory would be impossible.

Launching an all-out counterattack against Japan would have led to failure; victory demanded a carefully planned campaign. Industry had to gear up to produce war materials. Soldiers and sailors had to be recruited. Ships and airplanes had to be built, and pilots, seamen, and soldiers had to be trained. But eventually, by implementing a strategic campaign, the United States was victorious in the Pacific.

The Necessity of Job Hunting Skills

Fifty people from all levels of EMS work were asked about their career futures, and less than ten percent said they were planning to retire in their current jobs. A recent Gallup Poll surveying employee attitudes around the country found that one-third of working people expect to leave their current jobs within the next three years. The rapidly changing world around us means that almost everyone will change jobs several times over the course of their careers, and many futurists are predicting that in the coming decades people will change entire careers several times during their working lives.

Finding the job you want in EMS also demands careful planning and preparation. Because of the rapidly changing nature of the work world, experts say Americans today will change jobs more often than their parents did. This may be especially true in EMS, a new and rapidly evolving field.

The problem is, job hunting can be one of life's most stressful activities. Selling yourself to strangers means risking rejection. The whole process is ambiguous and full of game-playing. Consequently, you may be tempted to take the least painful and more passive approach to your job search—scanning the classifieds, asking around, and mailing off a few resumes—instead of actively pursuing the job you want. As a result, most of your time is spent waiting, and you never quite have control of your search.

But job hunting doesn't have to be a stressful mystery. While it may never be easy, you *can* take control. You can find the job you want and decrease the frustration of the process by being organized and systematic. Your

Job hunting can be one of life's most stressful activities.

job campaign will include the mission statement you prepared in Chapter Three and will entail five important steps:

- **Step One**—Clarifying the job you want
- **Step Two**—Setting parameters for your job search
- **Step Three**—Identifying potential organizations
- **Step Four**—Focusing on a specific job
- **Step Five**—Presenting yourself

Opportunities in EMS

Before working on your job campaign, let's talk about
opportunities in EMS. People often mistakenly believe that
EMS is saturated with workers and limited in opportunity.
But in reality, EMS is just beginning to open up. While
the profession barely existed and opportunities were slim
twenty years ago, the field has recently exploded. EMS continues to grow and diversify.

Traditionally, EMS meant working on a rescue squad,
on an ambulance, or in the fire service, but now there
are many more settings in which to apply your skills.

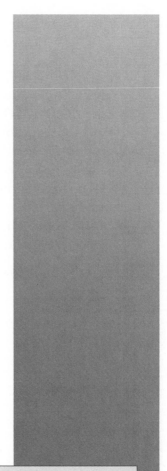

Unusual Opportunity in EMS No. 1

For medics practicing along the 800 miles of pipeline in Alaska,
work is much more than just another shift. These paramedics,
employed by American Guard and Alert, provide emergency medical
and general health services for the workers along the pipeline. They are
trained to be extended caregivers—to provide health exams, suturing,
and more routine healthcare, as well as ALS. The medics also work as
security guards between medical calls. They are often stationed in
remote locations and may work twelve-hour shifts for two straight
weeks before having two weeks off. The pay is exceptionally good, and
while on duty, food and lodging are provided.

Unusual Opportunity in EMS No. 2

Even in the idyllic setting of one of the world's busiest theme parks, EMS is needed. At Sea World in Orlando, Florida, a team of paramedics, EMTs, and nurses provides emergency medical care for the park's 4.5 million guests. Using specially designed golf carts to get around the park's maze of pathways and sidewalks, these providers must be prepared to treat everything from blistered toes and heat emergencies to mass casualty incidents. They must be trained in all the usual EMS skills as well as in water rescue and be prepared to stand by in some very unusual situations, like during a physical exam being given to a shark.

Wherever there's a potential for a medical emergency, there's a need for EMS. Furthermore, there are endless opportunities in education, management, research, publishing, communications, support services, and sales. Your options in this field are limited only by your vision.

To learn more about the occupational potential of EMS, you must first let go of your traditional views. Use your imagination! Begin reading professional journals—they will give you great ideas about what others are doing in the field and what you can do, too. Subscribe to as

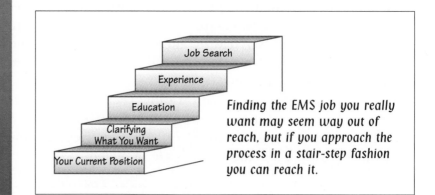

Finding the EMS job you really want may seem way out of reach, but if you approach the process in a stair-step fashion you can reach it.

many journals as possible, or look for them at a large university medical library. Browse through the articles, look at the ads, and read the news updates on how EMS is being practiced throughout the country. Write letters and ask for information.

Step One: Clarifying the Job You Want

Having clarified your purpose in EMS and written your mission statement, you now have a good idea of what you want. Now you'll need to translate your mission into a specific job or series of jobs.

Try This:

Go back to your personal mission statement for EMS. Read it over. What sort of jobs satisfy your mission? Don't limit yourself to the current market and what may be available in your area. Focus on your ideal job. Keep in mind your history, dreams, and values, but don't forget your talents, unique abilities, and special skills. Now describe that job with a title and responsibilities by completing the following:

The job (or jobs) I am looking for is (are) . . .

_____

_____

_____

_____

Along with clarifying the job you want, you must determine whether you meet the qualifications for the position. This process involves research, because there is little standardization of EMS nationwide and individual employers often differ in the qualifications they require for a specific job. For example, a street paramedic in one part of the country may need a good deal more training, such as ACLS or PALS, than would be needed in another area.

The best way to gather reliable data on qualifications is to consult at least five different sources. This may sound like a lot of work, but the more reliable the information, the better your chances of getting the job you want. Don't rely on your friends alone for information—there is a lot of misinformation surrounding EMS jobs these days. Instead, talk with people who are actually doing the job you want or who are intimately familiar with the position. Do

What Does It Take to Be a Paramedic for

New York City EMS. To be a medic for NYC-EMS, you will need to complete a paramedic training program and obtain certification from the State of New York. You will need to pass a test given by the Medical Advisory Committee and be physically fit for the job. The wait to be hired is about one year, and once hired, you will need to successfully complete the NYC-EMS academy's training program. There is not currently an EMS experience requirement, nor do you need to be a New York City resident.

Samaritan AirEvac of Phoenix. To be a flight medic for one of the nation's busiest flight services, you will need three years of ALS experience as a field paramedic, and you must be nationally registered and eligible for certification in the state of Arizona. You will need ACLS, BTLS, and PALS certification and, preferably, be an instructor in these courses. A written test must be passed as well as oral boards. Once hired, you will need to successfully complete a six- to eight-week training program.

Hennepin County Medical Center EMS in Minneapolis. To work for this busy 911 service, you will need to complete a recognized paramedic program, be certified as a paramedic in the state of Minnesota, and have six months to a year of ALS experience. A lifting test and health exam will be required. During your interview process, you will be orally tested on your medical and practical knowledge, and you will need to shine in a personal interview.

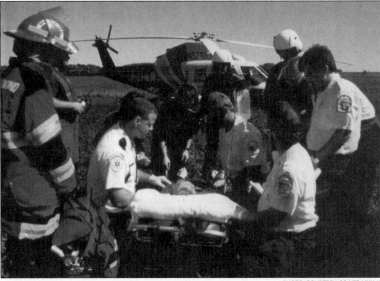

PHOTO COURTESY OF LIFE LINK III

a search of professional journals for additional information about qualifications, and contact organizations that have positions similar to the one you're interested in.

Let's say you're interested in becoming a helicopter flight paramedic. Place a call to a service you might like to work for, introduce yourself, and tell the person answering the phone that you are an EMS person gathering information about the qualifications of flight paramedics. Your introduction might go something like this:

> Hi. My name is _____, and I'm a paramedic student exploring career possibilities in EMS. My instructor, Ms. _____ recommended your organization as a quality flight service, and I'm interested in learning about the qualifications you require for flight paramedics. Can you connect me with someone who can answer a few questions?

You will almost always find people willing to provide information. You may be shuffled around or asked to call back, but eventually you'll find someone to talk with. If you are instructed to call back, though, ask for the name of someone specific. Having a name always makes calling back easier. Also, keep in mind that most EMS people enjoy talking about their work and organization as long as you remain polite, brief, and clear.

Once you've made your first call, don't stop. You may feel discouraged as you compare your qualifications with what you've learned, but push ahead. Keep in mind that you're just gathering data, and continue making calls until you have a pile of notes on exactly what is required for the job you want.

Try This:

Once you've talked with at least five sources about qualifications for your job, complete the following.

To qualify for the job I want, I need

Education/training: _____

_____

(List everything regardless of whether you have it.)

Experience: _____

_____

(Again, list everything regardless of whether you have it.)

Now highlight the qualifications you meet.

If you qualify for the position you want, go for it. If you need additional experience or education, don't despair. Many EMS positions require special training. Consider how far you've come, and remember that everyone is a beginner at some point in the process. Think about your dream and how rewarding it will be when you finally achieve what you want. You can make it through the next set of hurdles.

Getting additional education and training is usually fairly straightforward—just make sure the training you receive is recognized by the organization for which you want to work. Gaining additional experience, on the other hand, is not always easy. Begin by trying to clarify the specific experience required. For example, most flight services require that you have ALS ground experience. In this instance, then, you would want to find an ALS job with a service that has a good reputation, is respected by the community at large, and will allow you to sharpen the skills you'll need for a flight position.

There is nothing wrong with taking a less-than-ideal job for experience if it will help prepare you for your dream position. Consider it a stepping stone. One paramedic wanted to work for a big-city EMS service known for its high action and trauma. The problem was, the service required at least a year of ALS experience, which he didn't have. Instead of giving up, he asked the organization to clarify the exact experience it required and then moved to a suburb that had a fire department-run volunteer ALS service. For a year, he worked as a nursing assistant in an emergency department and responded with the volunteer ALS service. It was a hard year, but he finally earned the qualifications required and got the position he wanted.

One additional note on experience: There may be a way to get past an experience requirement. If you interview well, have a good employment history, and can offer something unique to the organization, you may be hired without the experience. Don't count on it, but don't be afraid to try. There are no hard-and-fast rules in EMS employment, and if you are persistent, you may be able to bend the rules.

Step Two: Setting Parameters for Your Job Search

Most of us would like to find ideal jobs that are close to home, offer everything on our terms, and pay the wages we need, but it's not always possible. The position you want may in fact mean a move, more education, less money, or a difficult work schedule. In deciding which

There is nothing wrong with taking a less-than-ideal job for experience if it will help prepare you for your dream position. Consider it a stepping stone.

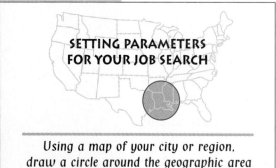

SETTING PARAMETERS FOR YOUR JOB SEARCH

Using a map of your city or region, draw a circle around the geographic area in which you are willing to work.

job to pursue, you will need to balance your work goals with other priorities and conduct your job search within those parameters.

Now return to your mission statement. What's really important to you? For most of us, work is a big part of our lives—we spend most of our waking hours working. Being happy at work is important. But what else matters to you? Balancing your wants and values will give your job search a clear focus and keep you from expending energy on positions that don't fit your goals.

Try This:

After reviewing your personal mission statement, complete the following:

1. *I am seeking a job in the following locations:*

   _____

   _____

2. *I am willing to move for a job under the following circumstances:* _____

   _____

3. *My job must pay at least* _____

4. *I am willing to work for less money if the position will take me closer to my ideal job.* ☐ *yes* ☐ *no*

5. *Other conditions I have for the job I seek (such as an unwillingness to work in a specific area, restrictions on shifts you are willing work, or anything else that would be important in clarifying what you will or will not do for a job):* _____

   _____

   _____

Balancing your wants and values will give your job search a clear focus.

Now that you've carefully considered the job you want, the qualifications required, and the parameters of your job search, take a few minutes to fully describe that job. Be as complete as you can. The more you put down on paper, the more focused and effective your job campaign will be. Here's an example from the paramedic student seeking a flight paramedic position:

> I am seeking a full-time paramedic position with a busy emergency ALS service. The service must respond to 911 calls and transports. The position must be in an environment that will help me perfect my patient care skills while giving me the experience I need for future employment as a flight paramedic. The service I work for must have a good reputation and be known and respected by the flight services I'm interested in working for. I'm willing to move to any location except the inner city or to a hot, humid climate. I need to make at least $24,000 per year. I am willing to work some overtime and extra shifts, but my personal health and time for myself are important.

Actually detailing the job you want is vital. You'll be tempted to find out who's hiring and what's available, but letting the market lead your job search will not bring you the job you really want.

Step Three: Identifying Potential Organizations and Jobs

Once you've spelled out the job you want and have a good understanding of the parameters of your job search, you will have enough information to begin looking at the market and identifying organizations that may hire you.

Begin by getting a map of the geographic area you are willing to work in. If the area is smaller than the map, draw a boundary line around your target area. Call municipal offices and hospitals and scan phone books, employment guides from the library, and computer bulletin

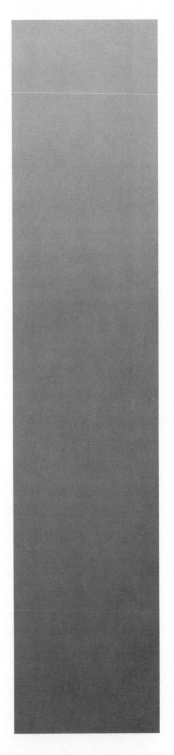

boards to compile a list of all the organizations that have positions fitting your job description.

Next, write the name of each organization and pertinent information on a 3x5 index card. You are now focusing your search on organizations you may want to work for. Try to answer these questions:

1. Does this organization have the job I'm looking for?

2. How can I get hired by this organization?

These questions require focused detective work. After all, finding out about organizations and how to get hired is like looking for clues. It involves thorough, detailed work.

Gather all the general information you can about each organization—name, address, phone number, director's name, number of employees, volume of business, and anything else that might be important. You can obtain most of this information from the organizations' marketing departments or even the receptionists. Write everything down on your cards, and don't stop until you have a good profile of each organization. This general data will not solve the puzzle, but it will provide the basis for further investigation.

Your best information will come from developing a network and contacts. The vast majority of EMS jobs are not found through the want ads or postings, or as a result of mailed resumes or applications. Rather, most jobs are found through networking. It may not seem fair, but in the real world of EMS, it's often who you know that counts. Therefore, success in your job search demands getting to know a lot of people in EMS.

A Pep Talk on Networking

Networking is the hotspot of your job search; it opens pathways to your goals. Unfortunately, many EMS people are turned off by the concept, viewing networking as "brown-nosing" and politics. One EMS job hunter put it

Most EMS jobs are found through networking.

this way: "Why can't I just be accepted for all the good things I do? Why can't I be hired for my skills and abilities? Sucking up to someone so I can get a job rubs me the wrong way." This view reflects an inaccurate and personal view of networking. Networking isn't about seeking personal approval from others, it's about building professional relationships to share information. Information is the lifeblood of your job campaign.

You build a network by meeting and talking with people. Throughout your training, clinical experience, and work, you will come in contact with people working in EMS. Every one of them, at some point, has been in the position of looking for a job. They may have insight and advice that can help you. They may know of job openings or be able to introduce you to someone who can lead to a job. Every person you meet in EMS can be a link in the network you build. Conferences, training meetings, and encounters in emergency departments can all provide new links.

Go out of your way to introduce yourself. When you meet people, take careful note of their names, and ask questions about them, their work, and their organizations. Try not to talk too much about yourself; just ask questions and listen. Also, don't mention that you are looking for a job unless someone asks. People may be turned off if they think you simply want to use them in your job search. Be honest, however, and say that you're gathering information about different EMS organizations and careers.

Try to act confident and relaxed when meeting people; don't act desperate, hungry, or worried. Be a good listener, and don't be afraid to ask people if they know someone else you should talk to. Also, ask if you can use their names when contacting people they may have told you about.

As you begin making contacts, you will develop your own style of approaching people. Remember that you're just asking for information, you're not trying to sell

"There's a network of helping hands behind every genuine success."

—Barbara Sher, *Wishcraft*

Every person you meet in EMS can be a link in the network you build.

Networking Rules

1. Don't wear out a contact; always end a conversation before it becomes laborious.
2. If a conversation goes well, ask if you may contact that person in the future. If so, write down his name and phone number.
3. Always thank a contact for his help. Following a short conversation, a spoken thank-you is fine, but if someone talks with you for an extended period of time, send a thank-you card or brief note. It will be appreciated and will help keep the door open for future contact.
4. Keep track of all of your contacts on 3x5 cards. Record the person's name, title, organization, address, phone, what your conversation was about, and the date of your contact. You may need help from this person in the future and will want to remember exactly what you talked about and when.
5. Keep in touch with your contacts through brief phone calls or letters. Too often, people do a good job of networking but fail to follow up with their contacts.

vacuum cleaners. If someone brushes you off or treats you rudely, shrug it off. Unfortunately, as in every other field, there are some arrogant, insecure people in EMS.

The real secret to networking is to keep your network alive. Talk with old contacts and continue making new ones. Try to make two new contacts every week and to talk with two established contacts every week. Though at times it may seem like a waste of effort, don't stop networking. You'll be surprised at what you learn from people.

Long-Distance Networking

If your search requires a long-distance job hunt, you'll need a different strategy. This sort of job search will require an investment in letters, phone calls, and travel.

Once you have a good concept of the job you are looking for, make a list of the states you would be willing to move to. Write to the EMS directors of each state and ask for a list of providers in your targeted area (e.g., ALS, BLS, air medicine, etc.). Using the list they send you, contact individual organizations employing the information gathering approach. Tell them you're calling long distance, and ask who you might talk to about employment opportunities. In this case you can be more direct about job hunting because, oddly, when you're calling long distance, your interest in employment is not usually perceived as a threat. Ask about employment, salary ranges, and requirements, as well as how often they hire. If someone seems annoyed with your questions, ask if there would be a better time or person to call. Most organizations are conscious of their image and will give you at least enough information for you to determine if you are interested. If nothing else, get the name and address of the director or personnel director, and then write that person a query letter.

Continue your search by calling a number of organizations in that area. Once you have enough data, plan a trip and make information gathering appointments with several organizations. It doesn't matter whether or not the organization has a job opening; you are simply trying to determine whether it is a place you might consider working. During your visit, you make contacts and gain more insight into how you might approach the organization for a job.

Remember, once you've made a good contact, don't let it slip away. Follow up with a letter or phone call. Letters can be especially effective in the long-distance search because they give the contact a chance to see your name in print. Just as in politics, name recognition is vital in the job search.

Another way to conduct a long-distance job search is by visiting an EMS conference in the area you wish to work. Conferences are great places to network. By simply walking the floor, introducing yourself to people, and asking

Once you've made a good contact, don't let it slip away.

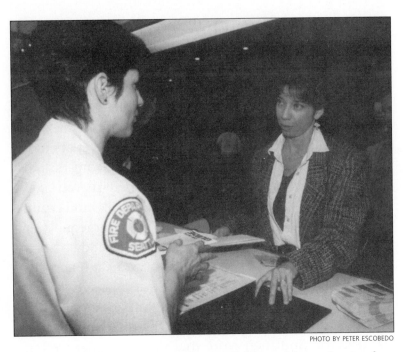

PHOTO BY PETER ESCOBEDO

Professional conferences are great places to build your job search network.

questions about EMS in that area, you will gather all kinds of data, including the politics of the region and who's who. Investing in a conference can be a very effective way to build a network rapidly in a place you don't live. It may actually save you money in the long run.

Step Four: Focusing Your Search on a Specific Job

Once you've gathered a substantial amount of data on all the organizations within your job search area, you'll have a good idea of which ones you want to pursue. Go through your 3x5 cards and weed out the organizations you don't want to work for. Do not eliminate the ones you are interested in but doubt you are qualified for. Now focus on these remaining organizations.

Once again, you'll need to put on your Sherlock Holmes hat and begin looking for clues about how to get hired at these organizations. First you'll need a contact or source within or close to each organization. This contact need not be a management person, and in fact, you may get more information from a non-management person. Hopefully, you have already made this contact through networking. If not, now is the time.

Your contact or source is critical. He will help you understand the inner workings of the organization, as well as what is currently happening and how you might get hired. Remember, you can let your contact know you're conducting a job campaign, but don't come off as desperate or hungry. Present yourself as enthusiastic about working for that organization, but also be patient.

Develop relationships with your sources and then build your relationships by investing in them. Show a genuine interest in your contacts as people. Take them out for coffee. Stop by with donuts or pizza. See if you can do a ridealong, or develop the relationship in some other nonintrusive manner.

As you work your network in each organization, gather data to answer the following questions.

- How did the past few people get hired, and was there something distinguishing about them?
- How did they position themselves?
- What specifically does management look for in a new employee?
- What can you do to prepare yourself for a position? Is there currently an opening?
- How often does the company hire?
- When is it planning to expand?

While you may never directly ask your contact these questions, as you learn more about the organization, you will uncover the answers.

There are different ways in which networking can lead you to a job. As you work your contacts, the path will become clear. You'll hear stories of how other people obtained their positions. You'll learn about unadvertised openings. You'll develop a feeling about how to prepare yourself for the next position. Eventually, you will uncover an opportunity you want to pursue.

Several years ago during a time when the EMS job market was extremely tight, many graduating paramedic students stopped working their networks and either left town or found work outside the field. However, one young man stayed at his job and kept up his EMS network, making polite contacts, calling old ones, and staying on top of things. But nothing seemed to be open.

One day, he called a contact at a mid-sized hospital ALS service to ask how things were going. His contact said the service had three paramedics out due to injuries and that it needed someone right away on a temporary basis. The paramedic was hired for a temporary on-call position. Within a month, the position led to part-time work. In less than six months, the paramedic had a full-time position. The opening was never advertised; this paramedic was hired because he exercised his network.

Another student took a job working for a non-emergency service doing wheelchair transfers. He used the position to develop contacts with ALS people everywhere he went. Before long, he became well-known as a friendly, helpful person. He looked for opportunities to chat with people, and occasionally would stop by a station to return equipment he had found in the emergency department. When the county service began its formal hiring process, he came with such high recommendations that he was hired over a large group of more experienced people.

As these examples demonstrate, even when seeking a position with a public EMS organization where the hiring process is highly structured and follows a regimen of testing, interviews, and callbacks, your network is still important. It will encourage you, give you a competitive edge, and show you how to shine in the process. Furthermore, EMS is a rapidly changing field, and by continuing

Your network will encourage you, give you a competitive edge, and show you how to shine in the process.

to cultivate your network, you will keep yourself open for future jobs and opportunities as your career develops.

Step Five: Presenting Yourself

Once you're ready to apply for a specific position, you will need to present yourself through letters, applications, resumes, and interviews.

Presenting yourself in the best possible light requires confidence in your qualifications and an intimate familiarity with what you have to offer. The best way to present yourself is by building an accomplishment-oriented resume. Constructing this resume can be a confidence-building process that will help you see exactly how much you've done and how qualified you really are.

EMS workers have often done much more than their job experience reveals. For example, many have done volunteer work, taught community CPR classes, organized training programs, and served in a number of different roles outside of their actual "job experiences." While most resumes highlight job experience, it may not be a complete representation of all you have to offer a potential employer.

Try This:

Accomplishment Worksheet

Make a list of your accomplishments both in and out of the workplace dating back to high school. List things that relate to EMS, but don't overlook your accomplishments in other areas. Have you organized something, taught a class, led a group, or researched a topic? What were your accomplishments in the jobs you've had? Did you coordinate a program, design a better way of doing something, or manage a team? Regardless of how insignificant the accomplishment may seem to you, write it down. Take a few minutes and list as many accomplishments as you can.

Presenting yourself in the best possible light requires confidence in your qualifications and an intimate familiarity with what you have to offer.

Most people are surprised at how many accomplishments they really have. Keep adding to your list as things come to mind.

Now you can move to the more traditional information for your resume.

Try This:

Education and Experience Worksheet

Detail your education, working back to high school. Include college, vocational school, special training programs, workshops, continuing education, etc. For each, include the school name and address, dates attended, the name of the course or program, and the certification you received.

School: _____
Address: _____
Dates Attended: _____
Program or Course: _____
Degree or Certification: _____

Now make a list of all the jobs you've held. Include the employer's name and address, dates worked, job title, and duties.

Employer: _____
Address: _____
Dates Worked: _____
Job Title: _____
Duties: _____

Once you've gathered all this information, you can begin writing your resume. Remember, the purpose of the resume is to give a potential employer a quick synopsis of your qualifications and to spark his interest in you. An employer is not going to hire you on the basis of your resume alone, but your resume may entice him to consider you for an interview. Therefore, a resume should be short, interesting, and professionally done. One page is usually enough.

A sample of an accomplishment-oriented resume for EMS can be found on page 82.

There are many different styles of resumes, and you can be as creative as you want. You can find resume examples at your library or bookstore, but first make a basic accomplishment-oriented resume and change it later to suit your taste.

Objective

Many resumes begin with an objective. The objective is a statement of your goal or intention, such as "To apply my education and experience in a challenging and progressive ALS position that offers opportunity for a diverse EMS experience as well as professional growth."

An Unusual Resume

"Of the thousands of resumes I've seen, only one actually influenced my decision to hire an applicant. This paramedic submitted his resume on a patient care report. His name, address, and phone number were listed in the space for billing information. Where it asked for physician's name, he listed a reference—his paramedic school medical director. And in the narrative, he described himself using the standard SOAP format: *Subjective* described his attributes—nice, friendly, dedicated, and hard working; *Objective* described his background, education, and employment history; *Assessment* described him as an excellent new paramedic and prospective employee; and *Plan* described his goals and objectives, laid out step by step.

His interview was just a formality. He got the job. Not every employer would like this approach, but speaking for myself, if one didn't, I sure wouldn't want to work for that company."

—Mike Taigman, managing director of The Fourth Party, a MedTrans healthcare management development company based in Oakland, California

While the objective is a way of letting the employer know exactly what you're looking for, most of the time your objective is obvious. Stating it on the resume will only take up valuable space, so you may want to leave it off, as in the sample resume. If you need to state an objec-

---

Resume of
James R. Robertson
3245 California Street #341
Storyville, Nebraska 68104
(402) 555-3452

Accomplishments

- Responded to emergency medical calls with a 911 BLS ambulance serving rural communities for two years.
- Developed an equipment exchange program for BLS ambulance services and area hospitals.
- Completed continuous quality improvement training for EMS managers through in-service program.
- Coordinated and taught first aid training program for YMCA summer camp adult staff.
- Founded and operated successful three-person remodeling construction business, specializing in remodeling for the physically handicapped.
- Completed advanced training in high-angle rescue and participated in twelve actual rescue missions.
- Researched and wrote paper on EMT stress in rural ambulance services during paramedic training.
- Participated in 1993 flood rescue efforts as EMT ambulance provider and triage officer during the Storyville rescue of thirteen flood victims.

Experience

- 1990 to present. EMT-D, firefighter. Storyville Volunteer Fire Department and Rescue Squad, Storyville, Nebraska.
- 1992 to present. Owner/builder. A&S Custom Builder, Omaha, Nebraska.
- 1990 to 1992. Driver. Roger's Trucking Inc., Omaha, Nebraska.

tive, you should do it in a brief, several-sentence cover letter, which will accompany your resume.

Accomplishments

When listing your accomplishments, do so in a manner that will demonstrate your diverse skills, self-motiva-

Education

Paramedic Certification—Middletown Community College, Middletown, Nebraska, 1993.

Firefighter 1 & 2—Nebraska Sectional Fire School, Lincoln, Nebraska, 1990-1991.

EMT Certification—County Medical Center, Bellevue, Nebraska, 1990.

General Studies—University of Nebraska at Omaha, Omaha, Nebraska, 1988-1990.

High School Diploma—Central High School, Omaha, Nebraska, 1988.

Certifications

National Registry of EMT-Paramedics #MP34567

BCLS Instructor

ACLS Provider

NFP Search and Rescue—Level 3

Interests

Nature

Hunting/fishing

Rock and mountain climbing

References

Available on request.

tion, and interest in the field. Choose accomplishments that fit EMS and are pertinent to the position you want. For example, if you're seeking a leadership position, be sure to show leadership accomplishments. If you're applying for an educational position, show teaching accomplishments.

When describing your accomplishments, use precise, but exciting action words, such as *coordinated, responded, taught, founded, participated,* or *authored.* Limit your accomplishments to the ones that best portray you, and remember that the employer is only glancing at your resume. Make it attention-grabbing!

Experience

In this section, you want to show a continuity of work—any EMS, healthcare, fire service, or community service employment will be important. List your current job first and work backward. Try to show a continuous line of employment. If you've had many jobs, list only the ones that seem most applicable to the position you are seeking. Don't go into detail about your duties in this section. The important things will already be listed in your accomplishments.

Education

Begin with the education that is most important to the job you want. Then list the rest of your education, beginning with the highest degree and working backward to your high school diploma. You can list college course work even if you haven't completed a degree, but be sure to be clear and honest. It's easy to mislead people about education, but the price for dishonesty could be the loss of a job.

Certifications

Here is a chance to list all of the cards and certificates you have earned. List your EMT or paramedic cer-

Remember that the employer is only glancing at your resume. Make it attention-grabbing!

tificate and number, as well as all your other certifications, such as ACLS instructor, BCLS instructor/trainer, PALS, BTLS, extrication-certified, firefighter 1, etc. Simply list the certification and number, if applicable.

Interests

This section is optional. Many EMS employers prefer short resumes that tell them quickly whether you're qualified for a job. They probably don't care much about your hobbies. However, if your interests are mountain climbing, water rescue, and flying, you might want to list them because they so closely parallel your professional interests.

Personal information should not be included on the resume. In most cases, it is illegal for employers to ask personal questions such as age, marital status, health history, etc., that do not directly relate to the job they are hiring for. If they have concerns about your physical abilities, they will test those during the interview process.

References

At the same time you compose your resume, make a list of three to five non-family references. Your network will come in handy for this. Use people who know you, are familiar with your work, and have good connections in EMS, such as a paramedic, an EMS supervisor, director, or chief, and a physician or emergency department nurse. An EMS instructor is also a good bet, as are previous employers. Make sure you contact all of your references and tell them you are conducting a job campaign and would like to add them to your reference list. Their recommendation may be less than flattering if they are caught off-guard and are contacted by potential employers without being prepared. In addition, references like to know what sort of position you are applying for and with whom so they can gear their recommendation accordingly.

Don't underestimate the importance of your references. Most employers check at least two references and

Don't underestimate the importance of your references.

want to hire people who come with sound, credible recommendations.

When drafting your list of references, include each person's name, title, employer, and business address and phone number. Print your references on a separate sheet titled "Professional References for (Your Name)." Keep this page with your resume, and be ready to hand it out at your interview or when you submit a resume for a specific job. Don't give it out if you are simply leaving a resume for someone to look over.

Next, write a rough draft of your resume. Have someone else read it and comment on it. Be sure to have someone reliable proofread it. Compose it in an attractive, easy-to-read type font and print it on a laser printer. Remember, your resume is a snapshot of you, and you want to make a good first impression by presenting a very neat and professional picture.

Applying for a Job

While you can simply send your resume to the organizations you'd like to work for along with a brief letter of introduction, keep in mind that this is a very ineffective way to find a job. Such shot-in-the-dark efforts rarely lead to employment. Rather, it's best to follow the employment process outlined by the organizations to which you are applying. This probably includes completing an application to be kept on file. Follow up the application and continue to work your network.

When you hear about a possible opening, call the organization's personnel office to make sure your application is on file and up-to-date. If in doubt, send in another application and resume with a one-paragraph letter to the director or person doing the hiring. This will put your name in front of the director (if only for a moment) and demonstrate your interest in employment.

As you develop your network and people become

aware that you are conducting a job campaign, contacts may offer to pass your resume to management. Your responsibility is to have your resume complete and ready. Nothing is worse in a job campaign than suddenly needing a resume and not having one, so always keep an updated one handy.

Sample Cover Letter

When sending a resume to a prospective employer, always include a brief cover letter that states your purpose and generates interest in some of your accomplishments. If this is a cold contact, always state that you will be following up with a phone call—and then make sure you do.

26 Windsor Lane
Anytown, Maryland 21219

Mr. David Johnson, Director
ABC Ambulance
12664 Medical Drive
Another Town, Maryland 21224

Dear Mr. Johnson:

I recently graduated second in my paramedic class at St. Luke's Medical Center and am interested in a paramedic position with ABC Ambulance. Ms. Rutler, my paramedic instructor, recommended your organization and suggested I contact you. Some of my accomplishments that may interest you are

• Four years of emergency BLS ambulance experience
• Instructor and coordinator for community CPR and first aid program
• Associate degree in health science from Anytown Community College

I have enclosed a resume for your review and would welcome an opportunity to discuss positions within your organization. I will call you within the week. Thank you for your time and consideration.

Sincerely,

Alice Loring

Occasionally, you will get an opportunity to sit down with a manager and talk about employment. When this happens, be sure to show interest, and leave a resume with that person. Even if there is no opening, you will leave a good impression and the manager will be familiar with your name.

Once you've applied for a job, be patient. Employers rarely make decisions when they say they will. If they haven't told you when a decision will be made, you may call the personnel office and simply ask when it will be made. Don't expect any more information. Most employers don't appreciate being bothered by impatient applicants.

Interviewing

The day will finally come when you are called for an interview. This will be your chance to demonstrate why you should be hired over the fifty or so other applicants. You'll finally get to speak directly to a person who can make decisions.

Interviewing can be very stressful—fear of the unknown tends to make us uneasy. You can approach your interview with confidence if you've done your research and practiced answering and asking questions.

Research

To interview well, you must have detailed information about the organization you are interviewing with. Go back to your 3x5 cards on the organization. How much do you know about it? What is the exact scope of services it offers? How many employees does it have? How many calls does it respond to each month? What are its standing orders? What is the relationship between this organization and the community? What accomplishments has this organization made in the past five years? Have there been any recent advances or setbacks?

One paramedic's recent interview experience shows

> You can approach your interview with confidence if you've done your research and practiced answering and asking questions.

the value of research. As he sat down, the employer asked him how he thought he would fit into the organization's current climate. The organization was a hospital-based ALS service that had just been purchased by a large HMO. The purchase had been covered by all the local newspapers and talked about throughout the EMS community. The paramedic had not bothered to do any research and had no clue what the employer meant by the "current" climate. Needless to say, he didn't know how to respond, and he wasn't hired. Learn everything possible about the organization interviewing you.

Question Preparation

Next, you'll want to prepare a list of questions you may be asked and plan your answers. It's difficult to know how the interviewer will approach you. Some interviews will be highly formal and structured, while others will be more casual. You must be prepared for either tack.

Possible Interview Questions

1. Tell me about yourself.
2. What brings you to EMS work?
3. What attracts you to this job and this organization?
4. Where do you see EMS going in the near future?
5. What are the most satisfying aspects of EMS work to you?
6. What are your strengths?
7. What are your weaknesses?
8. Tell me about some of your accomplishments in life.
9. Tell me about your greatest mistake.
10. What are your long-range goals in EMS?
11. How do you get along with other people?
12. How would former employers describe you?
13. How do your education and experience relate to this job?
14. How do you handle conflict?

Despite a long list of questions they may ask, all interviewers are essentially looking for the answer to three basic questions: Why do you want to work in this organization? What can you do for this organization? What kind of person are you?

1. Why do you want to work in this organization? This is where your research will come in handy. The interviewer wants to know how much you know about the organization and why you want to work there. Do you value all the great things going on in the organization, and is this a place you plan to serve loyally? The answer to these questions can come honestly from your entire job search. You may answer by saying, "I have a strong interest in working for this organization because of _____ and _____ _____. I am particularly interested in this organization because I excel in _____ and _____." If you've done a thorough job of researching the organization, you will have no trouble filling in the blanks.

2. What can you do for this organization? In this question, the employer wants to know if you can be an asset to the organization. How can you help it accomplish its goals? What specific talents, skills, and experience do you offer? Considering the current trends in EMS and the organization, how can you be an asset? This is where you want your abilities and knowledge in EMS to shine. Let them know how you can meet their current needs. Tell about your ability to provide good patient care, work odd shifts, and be

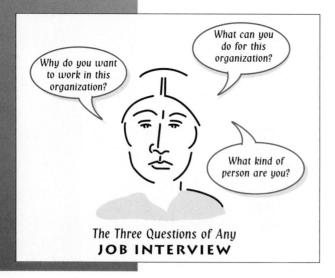

The Three Questions of Any
JOB INTERVIEW

available on short notice. Speak of your willingness to take on extra projects and how your past experience may be useful.

3. **What kind of person are you?** Here the interviewer will try to uncover reasons why the organization should or should not hire you. Your appearance, your attentiveness, your passivity or arrogance, your enthusiasm, and your general attitude will all influence his opinion. Go in with a positive self-image and present yourself in a manner that your research says the employer will appreciate. Dress professionally and be on time. Practice your questions and answers so you can leave some of your fear at home.

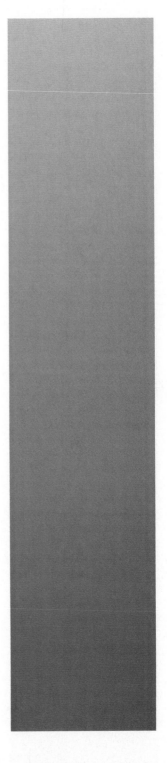

Try This:

In preparing for your interview, write out the answers to the three questions we just talked about. After writing detailed answers, take a stack of 3x5 cards. Write down ten questions from the list on page 89 and any others you think might be asked. Write one question per card. Go over the questions and think through your answers.

When preparing for your interview, don't forget to prepare several questions to ask the interviewer. For example, you may ask

- What would you say is the most challenging aspect of this position for a new medic?
- What are some of your organization's short- and long-term goals?
- If you hire me for this position, what criteria will you be using to assess my success?

The answers to these questions will help you determine whether the job is in line with your goals and whether you believe you can be successful in the position.

Try This:

The most valuable preparation for the interview comes from actually rehearsing the interview with another person. Find someone who will play the role of interviewer and ask you the questions from your cards. Your first time answering these questions will be rough (that's why you're practicing), but by the third or fourth rehearsal you will begin to feel comfortable and relaxed. Most people neglect to practice and wind up fumbling in the interview. Every good performance demands practice.

In addition to the questions, many EMS employers will give you a medical or rescue scenario with a potential conflict that has a hidden issue of patient care, loyalty to the organization, or personal leadership. You'll be asked how you would handle the situation. Here's one example:

> You've responded to a call at an expensive supper club for a woman who has dislocated her patella and is in severe pain. Before you can thoroughly assess the patient, a man in a suit claiming to be a doctor steps forward, interrupts your exam, identifies himself to the woman, and tells her he can relocate her patella without her having to go to the hospital. He is very assertive and has acknowledged your presence only to mention your medical director by name. What would you do?

Don't be fooled into thinking there is a wrong or right answer—there isn't. The interviewer simply wants to see how you would handle such a situation. Confidently list your priorities, mentioning that you are first and foremost concerned about the patient. Be sure you mention the need to represent the organization well and the need to make things at the scene smooth and professional. The interviewer is interested in your ability to think broadly, not have tunnel vision, and make the organization look good. Have a friend make up a few scenarios and practice.

Job Offers

It may seem like a long way off, but your interviews will eventually lead to job offers. When an offer is made, consider it carefully and make certain it's the job you want. Most employers will give you several days to consider an offer.

Beware of an offer that comes fast and demands an immediate answer, especially if the job requires a relocation or some other investment. Unfortunately, some EMS organizations take advantage of people, perhaps hiring them with false promises. Several medics recently told of responding to an offer and moving across the country for a job that had been portrayed as a 911 emergency ALS position. Once they began, they discovered the service was not a primary 911 emergency service and was used only as a backup to another service. Their twelve-hour shifts were filled with back-to-back routine transfers, and they rarely used their skills. They had failed to check things out and were forced to work in a less-than-desirable situation until they could afford another move.

Generally, you do not have much bargaining power in an entry-level EMS position. While pay scales are usually fixed, you may be able to discuss other job issues, such as hours, start dates, or how experience relates to the pay scale, as long as you remain calm and straightforward.

No Offers and Perseverance

Following the job search guidelines offered in this chapter will not guarantee success in EMS, but it will certainly improve your chances. EMS organizations can be fickle in their hiring. If you fail to land a job in the organization you want, regroup and try again, or try a different organization. Keep in mind that not being

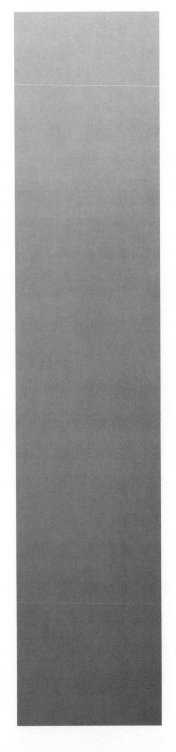

"Nothing in the world can take the place of persistence. Talent will not; nothing is more common than unsuccessful men with talent. Genius will not; unrewarded genius is almost a proverb. Education will not; the world is full of educated derelicts. Persistence and determination alone are omnipotent."

—Calvin Coolidge

Persistence is the most important virtue in job hunting.

offered a job is not a statement about your worth, value, or potential.

Nearly any person who truly wants a career in EMS can find work. Some have to work harder than others to find a position and some have to broaden the parameters of their search, but eventually they find that job. Remember, you create your own success.

You can learn something from every job you pursue. Consider every interview and inquiry a learning experience. We began this chapter by talking about World War II. In the early stages of the war, the United States lost more than it won. But eventually, lessons were learned, and the campaign was successful.

Persistence is the most important virtue in job hunting. Don't give up and don't accept the story that no one is hiring. This business is in a constant state of change. People quit, get injured, and are promoted all the time. Focus on what you want and continue networking and talking with others. Inactivity is a death blow to your job search. Find other EMS people who are conducting a job campaign, and get together and encourage each other. There's enough work for everyone, and sharing information will help you persevere.

Summary

✔ Finding the job you want in EMS demands careful execution of a plan.

✔ There are many diverse career and job opportunities in EMS.

✔ Conducting a successful job search and campaign includes five sequential steps:

1) Clarify the kind of job you are looking for and its qualifications.

2) Set parameters for your job search—what are your limits?

3) Identify organizations and specific positions through networking.

4) Focus your search on a specific job.

5) Present yourself on paper and in person.

✔ Recognize a good offer and persevere through the process.

Suggested Reading

Guerrilla Tactics in the Job Market (revised), by Tom Jackson (Bantam Books, New York, 1991). Considering the difficulties of the EMS job market, this book will stimulate some creative thinking toward getting that elusive job.

JEMS "August Career Supplement." Every year *JEMS* publishes a guide to EMS careers in its August issue. This guide is a great place to get ideas about education, careers in EMS, and how to further yourself in the field. It lists training institutions and profiles people who are doing unusual things in EMS. If you are conducting a career search, go through the last five editions of this tool for ideas.

Medical 911: The EMS Information Sourcebook (Jems Communications, Carlsbad, California, 1994). This reference book is a comprehensive collection of EMS information. It lists EMS agencies and organizations, consultants, attorneys, literature, reports, studies, books, journals, audiovisual and computer materials, and EMS products and services. In short, it is an essential resource for the EMS professional.

What Color Is Your Parachute: A Practical Guide for Job-Hunters & Career Changers, by Richard Nelson Bolles (Ten Speed Press, Berkeley, California, 1994). This annual guide is one of the most popular of its kind. More than five million people have purchased this book to assist them in their job searches. The author's common-sense approach will help you through all phases of a job search, including figuring out exactly what that job should be.

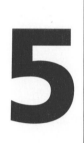Starting Right

Well begun is half done.
—Anonymous

One cold, dark Saturday night, my partner and I responded to a head-on collision on a busy two-lane highway. Arriving at the scene, we pulled a pale young woman from behind a bent steering wheel. She was breathing, but I could not palpate a radial pulse. I ran back to the rig for a pair of antishock trousers. The situation was urgent, and instead of taking the time to open up the trousers and quickly check them over, I simply grabbed one end and with the help of a bystander pulled them under the woman as we slid her onto a long backboard. We secured a chest strap, and while my partner worked at the patient's head, I tried to wrap and secure the trousers. But something was wrong. The Velcro was not where it was supposed to be. The trousers were on upside down.

Such mistakes are common when you're in a hurry, when you're excited, and when you don't take that extra moment to start a procedure correctly. The same is true with a new job. Starting a new job can be exciting, but often we are in such a hurry to get going that we miss the details of starting right. How you begin a new job is an important part of creating success in EMS.

Almost half of Keith Neely's paramedic novel *Street Dancer* deals with a paramedic's start at a new job. The paramedic, Danny, who is hired to work for Denver General's EMS department, wants to be a seasoned, respected medic the moment he starts the job. He wants to jump in the rig and handle anything the streets throw at him. But he quickly learns that starting right takes more than a few days on the job.

The "New Guy"

Starting right means giving yourself every possible opportunity and advantage to create success in your new job. Starting right means setting aside your assumptions about being new and giving yourself the chance to experience what your new position will require of you.

In EMS, there is no substitute for experience. No matter how much you know, how much you've practiced, or how much you've studied, nothing compares with actually doing the work. Most of us are extremely uncomfortable in a new position. We hate the label "new guy." We even associate being new with being incompetent, amateurish, or unprepared.

Because no one in emergency work wants to be known as the rookie, EMS workers try to shed the label as soon as possible. They want to be off probation and on their own while being recognized as fully qualified and capable of doing the job. Because they do this too soon, they're not prepared to do the job. Many EMS workers do not recognize the importance of starting right—they never gain the confidence and comfort level necessary for daily success.

Surrendering to the Role

To start right, you first have to deal with the discomfort of being new. When we're born, we are endowed with

"If you don't get off on the right foot, you're screwed. You can only learn so much from a training book and then you've got to do it—but you've got to do it right. If you don't get it in the beginning, then years later you'll still be fumbling on the big calls. You won't be any good if you're getting lost or still don't know the protocols. Confidence comes from doing things right in the beginning. This work is fun if you start off doing it right."

—A field training officer

In EMS, there is no substitute for experience.

"A journey of a thousand miles must begin with a single step."

—Chinese proverb

The secret to starting right is in giving yourself permission to be new and in surrendering to the role of being new.

great potential, but no experience. Throughout our lives, we are constantly learning new things and gaining experience. As babies, we are new to walking and talking. As teenagers, we are new to driving, working, and the opposite sex. In adulthood, we are new to the experiences of family, careers, and aging. Being new is a natural process of living.

Being new to something is a signal that growth and learning are taking place. When you experience something new, whether it's a job, a relationship, or a new vacation destination, you are presented with an opportunity for exciting stimulation and growth. You can choose to view being new as an opportunity or a burden.

The secret to starting right is in giving yourself permission to be new and in surrendering to the role of being new. To surrender means to stop fighting. Instead of rejecting the "new guy" label, embrace it. View being new as a positive experience.

Several years ago, I was a paramedic in specialized EMS transport where we provided interfacility ground and air transportation for critical care patients. With years of paramedic experience, I started the job feeling resistant to the idea of being new and submitting to the orientation. I was experienced in ambulance work and thought I could bypass the learning period. Then I had my first call.

We were called to transport a critical cardiac patient from a small rural hospital to the University of Minnesota. At the rural hospital, I suddenly found myself confronted with central IV lines with multiple drips, hemodynamic monitoring, and a ventilator. I was out of my league, but I tried to pretend I knew what was going on. I wanted to show my co-workers what I could do. After fumbling about for a few minutes, I finally had to let the other members of the transport team take over. I stood back and watched. It was very different from street work.

I hated being new, but I had a great desire to do the

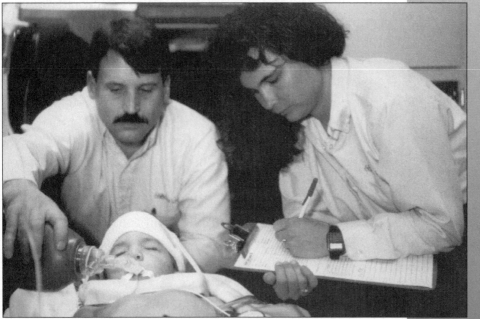

PHOTO COURTESY OF LIFE LINK III

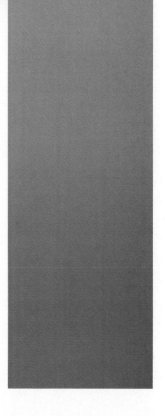

work, so I surrendered to the role of being new. To my surprise, once I let go of my ego and accepted that I was new, I really began to enjoy getting the experience I needed.

When you give yourself permission to be new, you put yourself in a learning mode, which allows you and those around you to contribute to your experience-gathering. At certain restaurants, the new waitresses and waiters wear badges that say "In Training." Some of them seem embarrassed to be recognized as being new, but it actually gives them an advantage: They have permission to be beginners at their jobs both with their customers and their co-workers. They are allowed to make mistakes. This is not to suggest that you wear an "In Training" badge in EMS, but post it in your mind and surrender to the role of being new.

In *Street Dancer*, Danny responds to his first gunshot call and discovers his training has not prepared him for the reality of the situation. The victim has been shot in the chest, and the entire scene is full of chaos. As the victim is lifted into the ambulance, he breathes his last breath. Danny suddenly finds himself in the back of the rig with a cop working a trauma arrest. He tries to start an IV, but the veins are flat. He's not sure what else to do, and his lack of experience becomes obvious. Then, to Danny's surprise, the cop doing CPR unexpectedly announces that he's a rookie just out of the police academy and is not prepared for the situation. Because of the cop's admission, the pressure on Danny seems to ease. He realizes that being new is something everyone experiences, and as he continues to look for a vein, he admits to the cop that he, too, is a rookie.

By admitting that you are new, you'll soon discover that your performance anxiety will ease. You will be able to gain the experience you need to achieve success in your work.

The New Job Orientation

In an ideal world, every new job would begin with a comprehensive, friendly orientation. But this is not an ideal world, and all EMS orientations are not created equal. Over the past few years, many EMS employers have begun to

---

A Typical Paramedic Orientation Checklist

- Tour of stations, dispatch, and central supply
- Orientation to rigs and equipment
- Introduction to policies and procedures manual
- Review of uniform policy
- Overview of service area and maps
- Tour of major streets and routes to hospitals
- Review of standing orders
- Demonstration of radios and radio procedure
- Overview of schedule and time cards

do a much better job with new employee training, but orientations can still be unpredictable. Some will last for months, with a field training officer evaluating every step of your development. Others will simply show you to the ambulance and send you out on calls with no training whatsoever. Even when thorough orientations are attempted, they are often cut short due to scheduling shortages, unexpected events, or poor planning.

Unfortunately, you cannot expect the EMS organization to give you a good start. Furthermore, don't assume that a formal orientation will fully prepare you for the job. Starting right and creating success in EMS demands that you start yourself off right by identifying what you really need to know and finding a mentor who can help you get the experience you need.

What You Need to Know

As you start your new job, you may at first be overwhelmed by being new. On your first day, you'll struggle to remember people's names, not to mention trying to remember where each piece of equipment in the ambulance is kept or what the fastest routes to the hospitals are. On your second or third day, things will not seem quite so foreign. Slowly, you'll begin to remember who people are and where things belong.

During your first few days on the job, consider yourself an observer. You can only absorb so much at once, so try to grasp the overall operation and what seems most important to the job. Observe how calls are dispatched, how the medics contact medical control, where the equipment and medications are kept, and some of the local geography. At that point, step back and ask yourself, "What do I really need to know to do this job well?" Think about the job and the basic duties you need to master. What are the operational procedures for going on a call, caring for a patient, and delivering a patient to the hospital?

During your first few days on the job, consider yourself an observer.

Consider such things as talking on the radio, maintaining supplies, and getting to your destination.

One way to determine what you need to know is to consider the things that cause you the most concern. When I took the job as a critical care transport paramedic, there was too much to learn all at once. The organization provided a good orientation, but I was still very uncomfortable with the things I didn't know. I was particularly worried about driving and getting lost, but I was also intimidated by certain pieces of complicated, unfamiliar equipment.

To deal with my uneasiness, I made a list of things I needed to know. Interestingly, I noticed that my list was quite different from the orientation check list the company provided. What may be simple for someone else may be just the thing that causes you the most concern. One paramedic may be terrific with radio communications and patient care but may panic about driving. Another may not give driving a second thought but may be terrified at the thought of giving a radio report or learning a new set of protocols. You must assess what *you* need to know to do your job well.

Try This:

After several days on a new job, make a list of things you need to know to do your job well. Think over the things required during a call. Your list may include items such as radio procedures, protocols, hospital locations, etc.

_____

_____

_____

_____

Once you've completed your list, prioritize each item as to which is most important to learn first.

Transfer this list to a pocket-size, multiple snap-ring notebook. Enter each item from your list on the top of a notebook page, one item per page, with the priority items first. This notebook is the beginning of your "porta-brain," an important tool for learning and remembering what you need to know in your new job.

As you work, begin filling each page with information that will help you remember and learn the things you need to know. Make sure your notes are concise, readable, and complete. Use simple words and phrases. It may help to photocopy prepared materials to add to your list.

Developing your porta-brain is an exercise in organizing and gathering precise information to help you do your job. The process of gathering and then writing down the information for future use reinforces what you are learning. Also, because the notebook is a ready resource, it removes the pressure of having to remember everything on the spot.

Make a goal of working on several items each day, again beginning with the most important. As you encounter new things, add them to your porta-brain.

I still use my porta-brain. It goes with me on every call and has literally been a lifesaver at important times. It includes important phone numbers, radio frequencies, drug dosages, hard-to-spell medical words, an abbreviation of standing orders, a hand-drawn diagram of how to set up a ventilator in an aircraft, and direc-

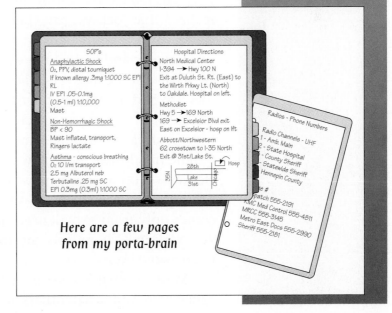

Here are a few pages from my porta-brain

tions to various hospitals. I also keep a list of all my calls during a month.

The Importance of Mentors

When I first began working in EMS, my lack of experience was obvious. Whenever a call came, I would run to the ambulance as fast as I could and then, with adrenaline surging through my body, I would attempt to talk on the radio. By the time I got to the scene, I could barely focus on patient care.

Then I met Joel Roen, a paramedic at the hospital where I was newly employed. I encountered him at the emergency department entrance as I was bringing in a man from a car accident who had fairly minor injuries. True to beginner's form, I managed to get worked up about the call. As the ambulance came to a stop, Joel opened the door, and I immediately blurted out that the patient had possible head, belly, and spine injuries. Having much more experience than I, Joel could tell that the patient was doing fine. "Hey, pipe down," he said. "There's no need to trip all over yourself." His rebuke was gentle and well-deserved, and I soon realized that Joel was just the person I needed to get me started on the right track in this work. He had been an Army medic and had all the experience that I lacked.

Over the next several months, I attached myself to Joel. He had a cool, confident attitude about emergency work. He knew how to detect a critical need and focus all his resources on keeping someone alive. He knew how to handle the drunks, and he was wonderful with children. He knew how to have fun, how to laugh, and how to debrief a bad call. Joel had the sort of street sense that comes only from experience. Much of what I know and do today in EMS reflects the things I learned from Joel Roen two decades ago.

Most of what we learn in life comes from personal experience and what others teach us. No matter what

> ### *How to Choose a Mentor*
> - **Do you respect and admire this person's work?**
> - **Does this person have good solid experience?**
> - **Is this person the kind of medic you'd like to be?**
> - **Can this person teach you what you need to know?**
> - **Is this person respected by others in the field?**
> - **Is this person willing to be a mentor?**

profession or career you are in, having a mentor—a trusted and experienced advisor—can be invaluable in your success.

Mentoring is a fairly new concept in most EMS circles. Some of the more progressive organizations will formally match you with a mentor. But most of the time, you'll need to find your own.

Keep in mind that not everyone who has more experience than you is a good mentor. Look for someone in your organization whom you respect and who represents the sort of EMS person you'd like to become. Approach that person and tell him that you admire the way he works and that you would like to learn from him. Even if you can't work directly with him, ask if you can talk about what is important to your new job. Most people will respond favorably to this approach. The relationship need not be formal as long as there is mutual interest.

Once you've identified a mentor, go out of your way to spend time with him. As with all relationships, this one takes an investment of time, but it will be well spent. Share your list of things you think you need to know and seek your mentor's opinion. Undoubtedly, he will give you a number of tips that will reduce your learning time. Tell him what you're afraid of, keeping in mind that he was new once, too. Review your calls with your mentor, and when you have a problem, talk about it.

One of the most important benefits of mentoring is that it builds confidence. Few things are as frustrating as a new EMS job. When I first began, I felt clumsy and was extremely critical of my performance. A run would go well, but I would only focus on how I could have done it better. Thankfully, my mentor was wise enough to support the things I did well and steer me away from destructive self-criticism. A mentor will help you focus on what really matters.

Learning the EMS Culture

There's more to starting right in EMS than just learning the "how to" of emergency work. A paramedic from Texas told of starting a job with a well-known EMS organization. His first day on the job he expected people to be friendly and welcoming. The managers were polite and professional, but the other crews barely greeted him.

"Some of them grunted a hello," he said, "but most of them treated me as if I didn't exist. One guy even came right out and said I couldn't ride on his shift until I got some experience. I sure didn't feel welcomed."

For a number of weeks, the paramedic didn't even feel like he was on the same team as his co-workers. People talked over and around him. They pulled stunts like starting to wash the truck with him and then disappeared, making him finish alone. When he tried to talk to people, they pretended not to hear him, but when he went on calls, they seemed to notice everything he did. From his radio procedures to his run forms, nothing seemed to escape their scrutiny.

This paramedic was experiencing an initiation of sorts. EMS seems to have a culture of its own. The culture varies from organization to organization, but every EMS group has its own particular way of acting, talking, relaxing, joking, and accepting new members.

Breaking into the EMS clan can be difficult for new-

Every EMS group has its own particular way of acting, talking, relaxing, joking, and accepting new members.

comers. EMS crews often become very close to one another because of the nature of the work, the tight quarters, and the need to depend on one other. They are usually very proud of their work and not compelled to accept someone simply because he puts on the same uniform. Consequently, the new worker is usually put through an informal, but very real, probationary period of initiation.

One EMS veteran explained it this way: "This isn't your average job. When you're in the middle of a rip-roaring run, you need to know if you can count on your partner. You can't do your job if you have to watch what the other guy is doing, too. And when it's all over, you need to be with people who can kick back and talk it over with you. Yeah, I'm pretty skeptical about the people starting out in this business today. I'm not going to trust someone 'til I trust them."

This initiation may go on for several months; don't take it personally. Eventually you'll be accepted into the group like everyone else, but you have to earn your colleagues' respect. Several guidelines will help you through this period.

Listen

Perhaps the most difficult part of being new is accepting that your co-workers have put you on probation. It's awkward. You'll try to end the probation by telling all sorts of things about yourself, talking a lot, and generally letting people know you're a good person and worthy of admission to their group. You'll be much better off, however, keeping quiet and listening.

Except for asking questions that pertain to your job, don't talk a lot. This may sound like harsh advice, but until you've proven yourself in action, most EMS people won't be interested in what you have to offer. They don't want to hear about your last job or about the time you

> *"Someone just can't walk in here and expect to be one of us. We've been through a lot together—we're a pretty tight group. We don't warm up to people from the outside right away. It takes awhile. They just have to sit on the sidelines until we get comfortable having them around."*
>
> —A medic

resuscitated three hungry children in the back of a Dodge station wagon in the middle of a raging blizzard.

If you're fresh out of paramedic school, you may indeed have current knowledge that surpasses that of your co-workers, but don't bring it up until you've proven yourself in action. Telling your new co-workers how to do something is not a productive way to start. If you have a lot of experience, it will be evident on calls and people will ask about your background. It's much more effective to *show* people how good you are, rather than to tell them.

As you listen and observe, you will slowly understand the culture of the organization. You will discover what's acceptable, what's important and who's who. In subtle ways, you will learn privileged information about the group and how it ticks.

Stay Neutral

A woman recently started a new paramedic position at an organization with a long history of management and labor problems. On her first day, several people cornered her and wanted to know if she supported the current director. The question surprised her, but she was wise enough to turn the question back to the questioners. She asked why they were asking. When she got an angry earful about the failings of the current management, she was thankful she had stayed neutral.

When you're new to an organization, people will frequently try to see where you fit in by asking your opinions about management, other workers, or certain procedures and practices. They may try to influence your thinking about the culture of their group. Staying neutral until you know more is very important.

You should also be prepared for people to try to draw you into their special group or clique. Again, the best approach for a newcomer is to be noncommittal and to focus on the things you need to know to do your job well.

> It's much more effective to *show* people how good you are, rather than to tell them.

Ethical questions can be particularly challenging for new hires. Unfortunately, not everyone in EMS performs with the highest ethical standards. During your orientation, you will undoubtedly encounter situations in which people will try to bend the rules, depart from protocols, or perform in a questionable manner. You will find yourself in a tough spot if you join in or if you report your co-workers to management. Handle these situations with extreme caution; you want to be accepted by your peers, but you also want to maintain your professional integrity.

Should you find yourself in an ethical dilemma, first talk with the people involved. If you can't resolve it at that level, talk with your mentor or get advice from a trusted outside source (someone in another organization, an EMS instructor, or a friend). You probably should not turn to management immediately unless the situation is of such grave importance that your own performance or the well-being of other people is in question. You don't want to be accused of doing something unethical, but neither do you want to jeopardize your potential relationships with your co-workers.

Of course, some managers may have a different view about how to handle ethical issues. While management would probably prefer that you report anything questionable as soon as possible, most medics agree that it is much better to try to work on issues with your co-workers. A reputation for "writing people up" or running to management will not make you popular with your co-workers.

Build Trust and Respect

As a new person, the most important thing that co-workers will want to know about you is whether you are trustworthy. I recently helped mentor a new paramedic who had gained a reputation at a previous job for being timid and unreliable. As I worked with her, she seemed quite capable in every aspect of the job. But none of her

The best approach for a newcomer is to focus on the things you need to know to do your job well.

> *"Whatever you can do or dream you can, begin it. Boldness has genius, power, and magic in it."*
>
> —Goethe

Respect and trust take time to build. They come from being honest, consistent, and reliable.

co-workers was willing to take my word for her; she had to earn their trust and respect on her own.

Respect and trust take time to build. They come from being honest, consistent, and reliable. Being new allows you the right to make a few mistakes, but you have to admit it when you're wrong. It is from your performance in these difficult situations that you will gain your colleagues' trust.

Building respect often means you have to hustle. The woman mentioned above earned the respect of her co-workers by doing far more than she was required to do. She identified the things she needed to know. She studied off the job and made a huge effort to learn everything she could. When a stretcher needed to be made, she didn't wait for help. When equipment needed cleaning and stowing, she jumped to the task. She accepted criticism and made a point of learning from her mistakes. Because of her attitude, people were willing to help her in the areas where she was weak. One of her goals was to become a respected part of the team. In a very short time she had earned the acceptance of the people around her. She had started right.

Interestingly, at the same time this woman started her job, another young paramedic with a different attitude was hired. This man expected to be accepted as soon as he put on the uniform. He had a cavalier attitude and assumed he was automatically equal to his co-workers. He often hid from work, had excuses for mistakes, and had to be prodded into learning the most basic tasks. Needless to say, his reception was not positive. People labeled him as lazy and unreliable. He did enough to finish his orientation and pass his probation, but his start left him far from being an accepted and trusted member of the group.

Beyond the Start

EMS orientations rarely end when the organization grants you full privileges to practice as a nonprobationary member of the team. It takes at least a year or two before one gains the necessary experience to do an EMS job well. As time goes by, you'll be able to assess if you've started right. The fearful things will seem less ominous, and you'll begin to have a relaxed sense of confidence about the work. Many of the things in your porta-brain will become second nature, and you'll have earned the trust and respect of your co-workers.

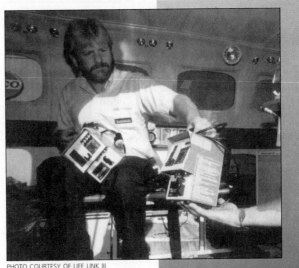

PHOTO COURTESY OF LIFE LINK III

One of the most important results of starting right will be the joy and satisfaction that come from being successful. Being new is a lifelong role. As you become comfortable with your EMS job, every day you'll discover new things to learn. This will help you create even higher levels of success.

Summary

✔ How you begin a new job in EMS will have a powerful influence on your success.

✔ Recognize that being new involves frustrations and the human need to find acceptance.

✔ Starting right in EMS means surrendering to the role of being new.

✔ Orientations in EMS can be unpredictable but you can create your own.

✔ Identify what you need to know to be successful.

✔ Find and use mentors.

✔ Learn the culture of a new position by listening, staying neutral, and building trust and respect.

Suggested Reading

The Magic of 3 A.M.: Essays on the Art and Science of Emergency Medical Services, by James O. Page (Jems Communications, Solana Beach, California, 1986). This book is included because a great start in EMS deserves a historical perspective. Jim Page is one of the founders of this business. This collection of his writings will give you a taste of the development and evolution of the EMS field.

Street Dancer, by Keith Neely (Jems Communications, Solana Beach, California, 1990). Although this book is fiction, it is a great introduction to EMS work. It shows how people and their ideas about EMS work are lived out every day.

Street Sense: Communication, Safety, and Control, by Kate Boyd Dernocoeur (Brady, Englewood Cliffs, New Jersey, 1990). Kate Dernocoeur's book is a great introduction to what you will find on the street. Compare the information in it to what you're learning in your orientation. This book is a huge resource and will be valuable throughout your EMS career.

Street Talk: Notes from a Rescuer, by Thom Dick (Jems Communications, Solana Beach, California, 1988). Thom Dick is a medic's medic and a great writer. He provides many practical steps for improving your work in the field. Just reading his book will give you a lot of respect for the pioneers in this field, as well as a glimpse of the real rewards of EMS.

6 Creating Daily Success

My philosophy is that not only are you responsible for your life, but doing the best at this moment puts you in the best place for the next moment.

—Oprah Winfrey

There is no such thing as a typical day in EMS. You may arrive for your shift one day and immediately be paged for a call in which you find a middle-aged man in cardiac arrest. You may clear from that run and start on a psychiatric call that turns out to be an angry, intoxicated teenager whom you sign over to her parents. The radio may be silent for a while, allowing you to return to your station, but later in the shift, you may respond to a nursing home to transport an elderly man with a cough. Still later, you may transport a dying cancer patient suffering incredible pain. No two days are alike.

Creating success may seem irrelevant in the middle of the EMS workday. After all, you go on calls and do the necessary work of maintaining equipment, filling out paperwork, and waiting. Yet, creating overall success in this work depends on your approach to *each* day.

A twenty-four-hour day is our most natural unit of

"Nothing is worth more than this day."

—Goethe

time. Each day is framed by the sharp contrast of day and night. A day is filled with the rituals of sleep, food, work, and relaxation.

In creating success in our careers and lives, we often fail to see the importance of each single day. We tend to think of success in terms of grand accomplishments, of having "made it," and of some nebulous time in the future when we will have conquered the struggles of life and achieved a certain level of comfort and security. But as we read in Chapter One, success in EMS is not a destination; it's a daily journey.

Several years ago, I was contemplating a career change and sought the advice of an older man who was very successful in business and in his personal life. I told him about my dreams and of all the grand things I hoped to accomplish in my life. I wanted him to tell me how I could be successful. His advice was simple: "If you want to be successful in all the things you've mentioned, start being successful today."

His advice seemed trite. I had been hoping he would

The Importance of the Day

The human body is synchronized to the solar day, a twenty-four-hour period of darkness and light. During this time period, the body goes through a cycle that affects such things as temperature, hormone levels, blood pressure, blood clotting, eyesight, mental ability, physical ability, sense of pain, digestion, bowel movements, and metabolism. Emotions, creativity, and thinking ability also rise and fall. This daily cycle is essential to human existence and profoundly affects one's perception of life.

impart a grand formula. I wanted to change my life, but not necessarily how I lived each day.

It took a few years, but slowly I began to realize that he was right. Success is not created in some glorious event down the road; it is a daily practice. If you want to assess your potential for a successful life, examine your daily success. After all, successful days add up to a successful life.

The Nature of EMS Work

The problem with creating daily success in EMS is the reactive nature of the work. How can success be created when so much of the work cannot be planned? In building a house, selling computers, or planting a garden, you can approach the day's work

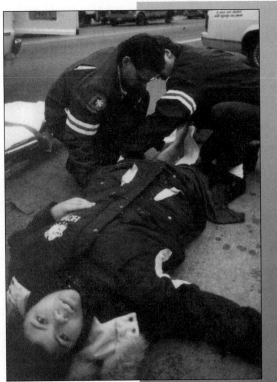

PHOTO BY MICHAEL KOWAL

by making a list of tasks to do and then setting out to complete the list. But EMS work is different. You never know when or where the next call will be, never mind what you will find at the scene. A call for help comes and you react. The radio crackles and you react. A set of symptoms is presented and you react. Those of us who do this work are called responders because we don't create the emergencies. We respond to them.

A great EMT or paramedic learns to react calmly and appropriately, but this coveted street skill comes only with practice and experience. Providers who learn to react appropriately to any circumstance or situation don't need to think about their actions. Their reactions become automatic. They see a shocky trauma patient and, without pausing, they slip into action, focusing their efforts on maintaining cerebral perfusion and getting the patient to

Successful days add up to a successful life.

Reactive Attitude

- Doesn't plan
- Waits to be prompted
- Follows
- Waits for things to happen
- Holds on to limitations
- Says, "I can't. I'm not allowed."

Proactive Attitude

- Plans even though plan may change
- Sees opportunity without prompting
- Leads
- Goes ahead with action
- Sees possibilities in everything
- Says, "I can. I'm going to try."

Success is not a reactive creation. It is a proactive creation.

the trauma center. Reacting calmly and competently is vital to good street performance.

While a reactive approach is necessary in EMS work, it can sometimes become a negative model for how we approach other aspects of our lives. EMS leaders frequently comment on how passive EMS people are in developing themselves and their careers. Part of the reason for this passivity is the reactive paradigm that comes from the work itself. Simply waiting for things to happen—and only being reactive—leaves one without much control and eventually creates a feeling of being used and victimized by circumstances.

Success is not a reactive creation. It is a proactive creation. While you cannot choose the next call, you do have choices about many things in your daily EMS work that can make a big difference to your success. You are more than a product of what happens to you. You can choose to create your daily success.

There are four important ingredients to creating daily success in EMS work:

- Planning for each day
- Acting in your circle of influence
- Seizing the moment
- Doing more than what is required

Planning for Each Day

Planning your day in EMS may seem silly. How can anyone plan emergency work? Granted, you can't plan the when, where, and what of your next call, but you *can* plan your approach to each day. You can plan your attitude, how you will respond to whatever happens, and the activities you will do when you are not reacting.

When thinking about planning your day, keep this in mind: If success is created, it is also planned. Anything that is created is actually created twice. Before a house is built, it is first created in the designer's mind. Before a road is built, it is planned.

The same principle is true in creating daily success in EMS. A successful day must first be visualized and planned.

Several years ago, an informal study asked approximately one hundred paramedics what they wanted from their careers and what made the difference between a good and bad day in EMS. The respondents said they wanted to have good calls, be independent in their work, enjoy the camaraderie of their co-workers, and be recognized for their contributions. These things don't happen by accident. Good calls happen only if you plan ahead and are ready to handle the difficult scenes and perform the necessary skills. Working independently and having time on your hands can be disastrous if there is no planning. Developing good work relationships and doing something meaningful for others is not a product of luck. The things we really want from this work take planning.

> *"The way you spend your days is the way you spend your life."*
>
> —Barbara Sher, *Wishcraft*

What Is a Good Call?

Every medic's definition of a good call is different. For some people, a good call is when everything comes out all right. For others, a good call is when they get to see something new, participate in a dramatic rescue, or be part of a big event. For most EMS workers, a good call is one in which they are clearly needed, their skills are challenged, and they have an opportunity to invest themselves in attempting to do something good for someone else. What's your definition of a good call?

Planning does not mean something complicated or time-consuming. Daily planning is accomplished by forming a conscious answer to the question, "How can I be successful today?" How can you be successful today, not tomorrow, not ten years from now? Finding a meaningful answer requires knowing yourself, revisiting your personal mission statement, and reflecting on what you want from your work.

When you fail to plan, you lose control over your day. The day ends up controlling you. Planning is not complicated. It involves reviewing in your mind—and sometimes on paper—how you will create your success for that day. Think about how you will interact with your partners and how you can productively spend your downtime reading, writing a letter, or doing anything that's not passive and that eliminates the heavy feeling of wasted time. You might plan something enjoyable for each day, whether it's laughing with your partners, pulling a practical joke on another crew, or taking a few minutes to enjoy the stars in the night sky. Keep your planning simple, but always make it a very deliberate, conscious act.

Try This:

Stop and imagine what a successful day in EMS will look like, and describe it in detail. What will your attitude toward your calls be? How will you respond to the routine, unexciting calls? How will you spend your downtime? How will you interact with your partners? How will you live a part of your life's dream today? What special things can you do at work that will be meaningful and consistent with your values? How can you enjoy today?

Hint: Review your personal mission statement for EMS and translate your mission into a daily plan.

> When you fail to plan, you lose control over your day.

Your Circle of Influence

In addition to planning, creating daily success demands an investment of time and energy. Unfortunately, we often invest our time and energy in the wrong place. People in this work often invest time in things over which they have no control. A favorite topic is the poor quality of management in EMS organizations. EMS people spend hours and hours critiquing their supervisors and leaders, all without much result.

In his best-selling book, *The Seven Habits of Highly Successful People*, Stephen Covey explains that successful people focus their time and energy on the things they can influence. They don't waste time on things they can't change.

As you engage in daily EMS work, you will be concerned about many issues that impact your work. Here are some of the things that might concern you:

- Drunk drivers killing innocent people
- A grumpy partner who treats patients poorly
- The condition of the equipment you use
- Back injuries and your ability to lift a stretcher ten years from now
- Improving your skills
- Always missing the "good calls"
- The future of the EMS industry
- The teen suicide during your last shift
- Healthcare reform
- Having a rewarding and satisfying day
- People who abuse ambulance services
- The state of your personal relationships
- The state of EMS management

Now draw a circle to represent your concerns and separate them from all the other things in the world about which you're not concerned.

> *"There is no use worrying about things over which you have no control, and if you have control, you can do something about them instead of worrying."*
>
> —Stanley C. Allyn

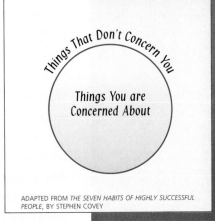

Things That Don't Concern You

Things You are Concerned About

ADAPTED FROM *THE SEVEN HABITS OF HIGHLY SUCCESSFUL PEOPLE*, BY STEPHEN COVEY

INFLUENCE

CONCERNS

ADAPTED FROM *THE SEVEN HABITS OF HIGHLY SUCCESSFUL PEOPLE*, BY STEPHEN COVEY

Of the many things that concern us, we can influence only a few. You might be concerned about the rising number of deaths of children by handguns, but your ability to influence that problem is limited. On the other hand, you might also be concerned about the impersonal treatment of people by our medical system. You can do something about that concern by beginning to treat people in your ambulance more personally. Our area of influence is smaller than our concerns; it can be represented by a smaller circle within our circle of concerns.

Look at this representation of concerns and influence. Where do you spend your time and energy? Many people invest a great deal of time and energy in their circle of concerns but not much in their circle of influence.

Several years ago, I rode with one of the busiest ambulance services in the nation. Many of the paramedics seemed angry and disillusioned. One young man had only been on the street for two years, but he seemed bored and cynical about his work. While transporting an elderly woman who was having trouble breathing, he was abrupt and unkind. Between gasps, she asked what would happen to her at the hospital. She was clearly frightened. "Lady," he replied in a gruff voice without looking up from his EMS form, "I don't know what they'll do with you at the hospital. My job is just to get you there. No one dies in my ambulance." His conversation with the woman was hardly comforting, and he provided no assurance or hope.

When later asked why he was so short with the woman, he reacted angrily: "Hey, if you were running nonstop calls around here, you'd be short, too. We're constantly hauling welfare cases and drunks. Management doesn't care how we perform as long as we don't get into trouble. They won't even buy us bullet-proof vests. No one ever thanks us. Most of our patients would rather beat us up than let us help them. They don't pay us enough to be happy and jolly with people. This entire EMS thing is a joke. You may get into the work because you want to help people, but you soon realize the whole system is using you. You can't change anything. I just put in my time and try to stay alive. This isn't Mother Teresa's work; it's just a job."

The paramedic was certainly concerned about many important things, but he was focusing his energy on his circle of concerns, not his circle of influence. He was reacting to things around him but not investing in the things he could change.

Successful people focus on their circle of influence. While they may be concerned about as many things as other people, they focus on the things they can change.

A few years ago, a talented man took a job as a quality improvement officer for a large and corrupt urban EMS organization. The company and its personnel were notorious for slow response times, poor patient care, and surly attitudes.

When asked why he took such a job, the man laughed and shook his head. "The needs are so overwhelming, and everything seems to be a mess," he said. "The whole system needs an overhaul." Then he became serious. "I've started working with the things I can change, and I don't waste my time with those I can't," he said. "Mostly I work on my own attitude and try not to let it become corrupt and fatalistic. I try to treat people with respect and listen to what they have to say. If I tried to fix everything that's wrong with this place, I'd become burned out in a week. I work on the things I can do something about."

Surprisingly, he did not burn out, become bitter, or become part of the organization's shortcomings. He didn't change things overnight, but slowly, people came to re-

> Successful people focus on their circle of influence. While they may be concerned about as many things as other people, they focus on the things they can change.

"Proactive people focus their efforts in the circle of influence. They work on the things they can do something about. The nature of their energy is positive, enlarging, and magnifying, causing their circle of influence to increase."

—Stephen R. Covey

spect him. He began to have a powerful influence. He made his success.

Try This:

Reflect on a recent day at work. Think about all the things that concerned you during the day. Hint: Concerns are often reflected in the things we complain about to partners and others throughout our day. Make a list of the many concerns you have in daily EMS work.

Next, underline those concerns you have direct influence over. Where can you invest time and energy regardless of your circumstances or the seeming limitations of your circumstances?

As you invest time and energy in the things you can influence, something surprising will begin to happen: Your circle of influence will begin to expand. Your influence will begin to touch other things—things that were previously outside of your circle of influence.

An old axiom says, "If you want to change the world, change yourself." As you become successful in the most basic of daily EMS tasks, you will notice that your influence is growing, and soon you will be influencing many things.

Seizing the Moment

Because of the unpredictable nature of EMS work, the opportunity to act in your circle of influence and create success will often be found in a fleeting moment, caught on the run.

My most successful and rewarding experiences in EMS have been flashes of opportunity that were totally unexpected and unpredictable. But because I was planning for success and operating in my circle of influence, those moments became great opportunities.

One sunny summer day, I responded to an accident scene in which a 4-year-old child had been struck by an automobile in front of the apartment building where she lived. The child lay crumpled in the middle of the street. As my partner and I approached, it was obvious that her injuries were beyond survival. She had an open skull fracture and her tiny body was broken and bleeding in numerous places. For the record, I checked for a carotid pulse while my partner retrieved a sheet. We carefully covered the child and, after talking with the police officers, headed back to the ambulance. There was nothing more for us to do. Just as we were pulling away from the scene, I saw a frantic young woman running down the street toward us. She was crying, and I realized she must be the child's mother.

"Stop!" I shouted to my partner, who was driving. He, too, saw the mother, but his response was different.

"We're clear," he said nervously. "The cops will deal with her."

"I want to talk with her," I said, getting out of the ambulance. The police had stopped the woman some distance from the child. They were trying to restrain her and keep her from seeing her child. As I approached, they quickly shoved the woman at me.

"Here's the paramedic," the cop said, giving me a look that said, "Get her out of here."

The woman was shaking and crying and demanded to see her daughter. I gently put my arm around her, introduced myself, and tried to move her away from the street. I went through the usual explanations about checking the child over and not being able to do anything. I told her that her daughter had probably not suffered and that we had to wait for the medical examiner before she could be moved or touched.

The woman's grief was profound. She seemed not to hear me. She was breathing with gasping sobs, and I had

"Carpe diem, quam mimimum credula postero."

(Seize the day and put as little trust as you can in tomorrow.)

—Horace

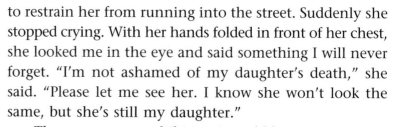

to restrain her from running into the street. Suddenly she stopped crying. With her hands folded in front of her chest, she looked me in the eye and said something I will never forget. "I'm not ashamed of my daughter's death," she said. "Please let me see her. I know she won't look the same, but she's still my daughter."

The woman was exhibiting incredible courage and an understanding of life and death that dwarfed my medical explanations. Instinctively, I knew she was right. So, contrary to usual practice, I led the woman out into the street, past the gathering crowd and to her little girl's crumpled body. I bent over and pulled back the sheet for the mother to see. She knelt beside the girl and tenderly wiped some blood from her daughter's cheek. She bent over and spoke softly to the child as only a mother can and then, as if tucking the child into bed, she straightened the sheet, tucked it about the little body and stood, signaling that she was finished. With tears streaming down her face, she thanked me and disappeared into the arms of several other women in the crowd.

It was a small moment, yet it was one of the most moving and gratifying of my paramedic career. The police officers later told me they would not have let the woman see the child and that they were grateful for my small act. Yet to me, it seemed I had done nothing at all.

On another occasion, I was transporting a scruffy young man who had threatened suicide and was on a police hold. The man was frightened and was clearly at a crossroads in his life. He asked what would happen to him. Would he be locked up at the hospital or would he be allowed to go home that night? I quickly explained the assessment process and the reason for a secured exam room. I saw him tense up at the thought of being in a psychiatric holding room; his eyes said, "Please help me, I never intended for my threats to go this far." It was a moment worth seizing.

I put down my EMS form and began talking to the man. I explained that even though his current situation seemed pretty awful, this trip to the hospital could be the beginning of getting some help and starting a new life. I encouraged him not to follow his fear, but to see the whole thing as a time-out, a time to get some help. I reminded him that he had done nothing wrong and that if he was honest with the people at the hospital, he could get the help he needed.

Nothing I said to the man seemed profound to me. In fact, I had completely forgotten the call until several years later. I was in uniform, purchasing fuel for the ambulance at a quick-stop service station when a success-ful-looking man in a business suit stopped me. I didn't recognize him, but he identified himself as the suicidal man I had transported and forgotten.

"Your encouragement made me see going to the hos-pital in a whole different light," he said. "I was so mixed up that night, but you pointed me in the right direction. Of all the things people said to me, what you said stuck with me. That night was the beginning of something new. I just wanted to say thanks." He shook my hand vigor-ously and walked away.

Without much effort, but by taking advantage of the moment, I had made a tremendous difference in someone's life. As I drove away in the ambulance, I felt immensely successful.

Seizing the moment need not always concern patient care. One Christmas day when my children were small, I was called into work unexpectedly for a mandatory shift. I had planned to be with my family and was angry that someone else had called in sick. The shift was to be spent at a fairly slow base with a paramedic I didn't know well. I was prepared for a perfectly miserable holiday.

When I arrived at work, I immediately began to com-plain about having to work on Christmas. With a twinkle

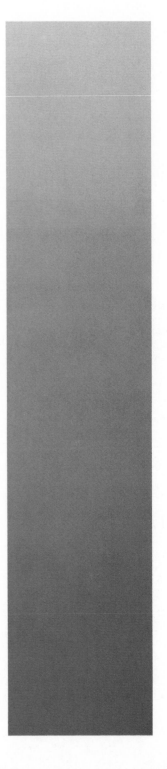

in his eye, my partner said, "Hey, this is Christmas. Lighten up. Let's make the best of it." Together, we created a holiday that in my gallery of memories has become one of the best. We cooked a scrumptious meal, invited several cops to eat with us, went on a few minor calls, watched Bing Crosby, and then met another crew and sang Christmas carols through the siren PA system. The shift flew by. When it was over, I realized we had created a truly wonderful holiday, all because we had taken the opportunity to make the best of what we had.

Success is planned, but the moment-by-moment opportunities come fast. They must be grabbed, or they slip by. Every EMS workday will present opportunities for success. By seizing the moment, you can create your daily success in unexpected situations.

Going Beyond What's Required

Professionalism is a term used frequently in EMS circles. EMS people are instructed to be professionals and act professionally, but no one seems to really define professionalism. In the modern world, the word has been used to refer to people who are specialized in some area or who can perform a specific skill. We often think of professionals as people who look, act, and conduct themselves in ways that are becoming to their profession.

Yet, professionalism is more than just a title and a way of acting and looking. Have you ever noticed that some of the best EMS caregivers are not necessarily the ones with the shiniest shoes or the slickest assessment skills? True professionalism is not about position or about how one talks or behaves. Instead, it is about how one values one's work. The real difference between a professional and a nonprofessional is not the color of the collar, but the attitude one has toward the work. The nonprofessional says, "I do this work because I have to earn a living. What do I need to do to earn my wage?"

True professionalism is about how one values one's work.

On the other hand, the professional says, "I do this work because the work itself is valuable. I'm glad you pay me because I need to earn a living, but the work itself is valuable to me apart from the wages."

Many people start their EMS careers with professional attitudes, but they frequently lose sight of the value of the work and do only what is required to earn their paychecks. Their value of the work slips away, and so does their sense of daily success and accomplishment. A powerful way of checking this loss of professionalism and success is to make a habit of doing more than you are required to do.

No matter where you work, there will always be a number of requirements. You may or may not agree with what you have to do, but exceeding the basic requirements will help create your daily success.

When we do more than we absolutely have to do, we make an investment in our work. Investing in our work is like investing in anything—the more we invest, the more we value the object, person, or work we are investing in. Doing more than is required is a subtle way of reminding ourselves that the things we've chosen to do have real value and are truly worth our time and effort.

Any job can become boring and less valuable. Recently, an airline captain revealed that one of the most common problems among flight crews in big jets is the loss of motivation and value for the work. While most people would consider flying one of the world's largest jetliners an exciting job, the job can become routine.

In the course of a busy EMS day, it's easy to get lulled into doing the bare minimum. But doing more than what's required of you is a wonderful way to reinvest yourself in your work. As you do more, important things begin to happen: You become better at the job you are doing because your skills and talents grow with use. You begin to feel better about yourself and your performance. As dis-

Doing more than what's required of you is a wonderful way to reinvest yourself in your work.

"If you resolve, beginning tomorrow, to put out more on your job than you're getting paid to do, miracles will begin happening in your life. . . . The most certain way to condemn yourself to a life of failure and tears is by doing only the work covered in your paycheck."

—Og Mandino

cussed in Chapter Two, a good estimation of yourself and your performance is essential to success. And as you do more, your performance will continually become better, which has a powerful effect on self-esteem and confidence.

If you only do the minimum, no one else may notice, but you will. Being successful is not about what others think, but about your own creation. Doing more than what is required is like spreading a warm blanket of success across your workday. You create success when you invest in the things you value.

I stumbled across the idea of doing more than what is required several years ago while reading a book by the motivational writer Og Mandino. I began following his advice on a daily basis in my EMS work and immediately noticed a change. As I began giving just a little more than what was necessary in patient care and in the routine chores of my work, I began to feel much more ownership and pride for my work.

When people do only what is required of them, they set themselves up for a narrow view of their work. Through their actions, they tell themselves that what they do does not matter and that their extra effort is inconsequential. But in the work of helping others, there are no small deeds. Just because no one notices the extra comfort you provide a cancer patient on a bumpy ride to the hospital doesn't mean it's without value.

Try This:

An unproven idea is worthless, so test out the principle of doing more than what is required. Reflect on three areas in your EMS work: patient care, interaction with co-workers, and daily chores (equipment, checking out rigs, paperwork, station duties, etc.). Jot down several things you could do on a daily basis in each of these areas that would take you beyond the requirements.

Patient care: _____

_____

_____

Interaction with co-workers: _____

_____

_____

Chores: _____

_____

_____

For a two-week period, apply the principle of doing more than what is required. Take note of your attitude about your job each time you do more, as well as at the end of each shift. As you invest more, see if you begin to notice any changes in your daily success.

The EMS people I respect most are the ones who invest themselves in their daily work and do more than the job requires. Many of them are not the most "professional" in appearance or presentation, nor are they always blindly obedient and loyal to their organization. But they all have a deep value for the work they do. They consistently go out of their way to do something extra for the people they care for and for the people they work with. Incidentally, these people are the ones who also seem to enjoy their work the most.

Creating daily success takes practice, but every day is a new opportunity to try again. Success doesn't just happen. It is a proactive creation. Every day will not be perfect. Start developing a powerful image of what a successful day looks like. Begin working in your circle of influence to seize those moments that will inevitably come. As you begin to string successful days together, you will discover that you have created a successful career—and beyond that—a successful life.

> Creating daily success takes practice, but every day is a new opportunity to try again. Success doesn't just happen. It is a proactive creation.

Summary

✔ Success in EMS is created not in months and years but on a daily basis.

✔ The nature of emergency work fosters a reactive approach to the workday.

✔ Success demands a proactive, rather than reactive, approach.

✔ Workdays in EMS *can* be planned.

✔ Focus your energy on the things you can influence.

✔ Success is found by seizing the unexpected moments.

✔ In doing more than is required, you will end each day with a powerful sense of accomplishment.

Suggested Reading

A Better Way to Live, by Og Mandino (Bantam Books, New York, 1990). Og Mandino is one of the world's best-selling inspirational writers, but his life was not always smooth. This book describes how, at the age of 35, Mandino was a derelict and ready to commit suicide. Mandino changed his life by learning to make the most out of every day.

Paramedic, by Paul D. Shapiro (Bantam Books, New York, 1991). New York City paramedic Paul Shapiro gives a good glimpse into the daily life of EMS. This book does not show EMS at its best; instead, Shapiro gives us an example of how daily EMS life can become addictive and difficult to manage without a plan.

The Seven Habits of Highly Effective People, by Stephen Covey (Simon and Schuster, New York, 1989). It's easy to see why this book has been one of the best-selling self-help books of all time. *Seven Habits* is one of the most important books

I've found for creating success in my own life. Half of the book is about learning how to develop yourself in areas such as time management and planning a future. The other half is about learning how to get along with people. Of all the books listed here, this one ranks at the top.

When All You've Ever Wanted Isn't Enough, by Harold Kushner (Pocket Books, New York, 1986). This is a great guide to making the most of every day. Harold Kushner is a rabbi who may not know much about EMS but knows what's important for creating success in one's life.

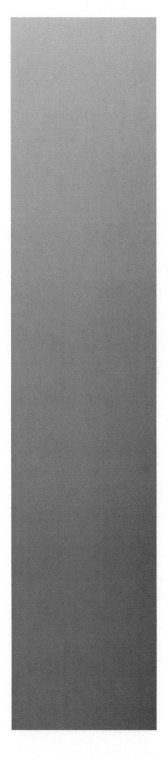

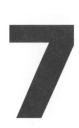

7 Success With Management and the Organization

The people who get on in this world are the people who get up and look for the circumstances they want, and, if they can't find them, make them.

—George Bernard Shaw

In commenting on why she liked EMS, a paramedic said, "I love this work because when I'm on calls, I'm in charge. I don't have a boss looking over my shoulder. I call the shots and get to see the results." EMS workers value the independence of their work. Skills are practiced outside institutional walls. There is the freedom of being in motion. There is the responsibility of making critical decisions quickly and independently in the heat of a crisis. Yet, EMS work is not totally independent. It must be practiced within the purview of an organization.

Developing a satisfying relationship with the organization and its managers may be one of the most difficult aspects of EMS work. EMS workers regularly report that their biggest source of stress is not the traumatic calls, the night shifts, or the dangers of the work, but the organization and management. Why is this?

EMS organizations seem to have earned the blame for

the way EMS workers feel about them. Many are poorly managed and underfunded and have unrealistic expectations of their employees. Many invest more in their trucks, radios, and medical equipment than in their staff. It's hard to believe, however, that the organizations alone are responsible for the poor relationship with their EMS workers. Much of the stress and frustration comes from the workers' incomplete understanding of their relationships with the organizations and how to make those relationships work.

Unmasking the Organization

When people first begin working in EMS, they often idealize the organization for which they work. Organizations sometimes represent themselves in an altruistic way; the new workers simply expect the organization to act accordingly. When the organization eventually fails to live up to the expectations, the employees' views of the organization suffer.

So what, then, is an organization? It is simply a collection of resources brought together to fulfill a very specific purpose. An organization will always work toward fulfilling its purpose, often to the detriment of other considerations.

Keep in mind, however, that an organization's actual purpose may be much different from its stated mission. For example, an airline may say that its mission is to provide fast, efficient, friendly service for its customers and a warm, supportive environment for its employees. But in reality, the organization's primary purpose is to make money and to be profitable. This does not make the organization dishonest—it means that it must balance its mission with its purpose and,

"They're always telling us about the stress we'll have in EMS from all the gory stuff. But that doesn't bother me nearly as much as management. It's management that makes my work difficult. If I go home from work frustrated and stressed out, it's not because of the calls. It's usually because management or the company is doing something screwy."

—A medic on stress

The organization may often seem like these theater masks, either good or evil, but underneath it is neither.

"An organization should function organically, which means that its purposes should determine its structure, rather than the other way around. It should function as a community rather than a hierarchy and offer autonomy to its members, along with tests, opportunities, and rewards. Ultimately, an organization is merely the means, not the end."

—Warren Bennis

when times get tough, the purpose will generally dictate how the organization reacts.

If the airline begins to lose money, it will react according to its actual purpose, laying off employees or tightening the budget. EMS organizations are no exception. Throughout the country, organizations have been forced to downsize and to become more efficient in order to fulfill their actual purpose.

The balancing act can be difficult for employees to reconcile. Workers grow disappointed when their expectations are not met. Recently, an ambulance organization demonstrated its primary purpose by instituting system status management (SSM) in an effort to become more efficient. The organization's primary purpose is to be profitable, and by using SSM it hopes to increase its loaded unit hours (the actual time paramedics are transporting patients). The new system requires the paramedics to work an assortment of odd shifts that start at various times of the day and night. In addition, the paramedics are required to wait and cover calls in their ambulances at street corner postings.

This change to SSM made the paramedics angry and bitter. They think the organization betrayed them and failed to consider their needs when it should have been primarily interested in the comfort and welfare of its employees. Yet, the organization has only acted in a manner consistent with its primary purpose. The workers' expectations are what have brought about the disappointment.

Many EMS workers expect their organizations to act as a parent acts toward a child—take care of them, value their work, and show concern for their future. It's not surprising that workers have this expectation. Historically, many organizations have fostered employee dependence. When my grandfather went to work for Fischer Auto Body fifty years ago, the company was very parental. It gave him a good wage and good benefits and provided for his future through advancement and retirement. The company said, "If you're loyal and stick with us, we'll take care of you." True to its words, Fischer took good care of my grandfather even after he retired.

Times have changed and, regardless of the impressions they create, most organizations can no longer afford to be parental.

EMS organizations often portray themselves as caring deeply for their employees, and many do. They provide fair wages, good working conditions, and reasonable benefits. But they are still bound to a primary purpose beyond their employees, whether it is to make money, provide a community service, or market a medical center.

In creating success, you must have realistic expectations of your relationship with the organization. What are your expectations of your EMS organization?

Try This:

Make a list of expectations you have of your EMS organization. What do you expect the organization to do for you? What do you expect beyond your pay and benefit package?

I expect my organization to . . .

_____

_____

_____

_____

_____

Now review your expectations. Are they realistic? A good way to assess how realistic your expectations are is to consider them in the context of the organization's primary purpose.

> In creating success, you must have realistic expectations of your relationship with the organization.

"Look, patient care is most important around here. But the truth is, if we don't pay the bills, you won't be taking care of any patients. So, you tell me what's most important."

—An EMS director

Try This:

Spend some time studying your organization, including its history and its leaders. Obtain copies of the organization's formal mission statement, values list, and guiding principles, if they exist. Then consider the following questions:

- *What is the stated mission of your organization?*
- *What are management's biggest concerns?*
- *Why does your organization exist?*
- *What is your organization trying to accomplish on a daily basis?*
- *What is the real mission of your organization?*

Write a brief description of what you believe to be your organization's true mission. Compare your statement with the organization's formally stated mission.

Consider the values of your organization. In its everyday practice, what does it value most? How do these values compare with yours?

A good look at your organization's primary purpose may reveal that you have more responsibility for your personal career success than you thought. You can't count on the organization to parent you. You can't expect the organization to pat you on the back, ensure your comfort, or guarantee your future. The organization is not responsible for, or ultimately interested in, your success.

Adjusting your expectations can be a rude awakening. As you can see, beneath the mask the organization is neither a shining prince nor an evil monster. Your relationship with your organization will be much healthier if it is based on realistic expectations.

Troubled Times

Every summer, my son and I go on an adventure in the Boundary Waters Canoe Area, a million-acre wilderness of lakes and forest between Minnesota and Ontario, Canada. The country is beautiful, the fishing great, and the opportunity for solitude endless. Each year, as the date of our departure draws near, we both begin to dream about how great the experience will be.

When the day arrives, we load our canoe with supplies and head into the wilderness, trailing fishing lines behind. We are soon reminded of why the wilderness is wild. Without exception, we always encounter some sort of unplanned trouble—several days of rain, an attack of mosquitoes, or a nighttime food robbery by pirating black bears. These troubles change the complexion of the adventure, sometimes causing frustration and anger. But we've learned that such troubles, even when severe, need not ruin the trip as long as we remind ourselves why we are there and what we want from the adventure.

As long as things go smoothly, your relationship with the organization will be easy. But eventually, like the summer canoe adventure, you will encounter some sort of trouble. It may be an issue of pay, a schedule change, or the growing feeling that the organization doesn't value your work. It may be a disagreement about a policy issue, a criticism of your performance, or a personal conflict with a manager or co-worker.

Such troubles can lead to some very negative feelings toward the organization and your job. You will try to work, but the nagging weight of the problem will color everything you do.

Dealing with an organization can leave you feeling powerless. The organization seems to hold

> *"If you have a job without aggravations, you don't have a job."*
> —Malcolm Forbes

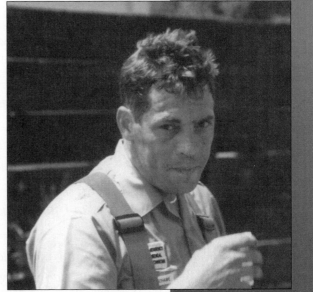
PHOTO BY JIM MALLORY/CONSULTING SYSTEMS, INC.

"Job security is gone. The driving force of a career must come from the individual."

—Homa Bahrami

all the cards. It makes the rules. It pays the bills. It even has the power to give your job to someone else. But you have more power than you think. The secret to empowering yourself comes in gaining perspective. On the canoe trip, my son and I cannot control the rain, the mosquitoes, or the bears, but we can assess why we're there, what we want from our relationship with the wilderness, and how we will react.

Perspective in your job comes from gaining a clear understanding of what you want and why you do what you do. Your personal success in EMS does not depend on the organization. When you find yourself in troubled times with the organization, stop and assess the relationship. Re-evaluate the job, your goals, your mission, and how it all fits with the organization's primary purpose.

Try This:

Troubleshoot your relationship with the organization. Answer the following questions using your personal mission statement and your description of the organization's primary purpose.

1. How has the organization changed in such a way that it is affecting my success? _____
_____

2. How has my mission changed? _____
_____

3. How will either the organization's change or my change affect our relationship? _____
_____

4. Can I still be successful in this organization? _____
_____

Answering these questions will help clarify your relationship with the organization during troubled times.

In completing the above self-assessment, you may discover some interesting things about yourself and the source of your frustration. Organizations do change, but frustration more often comes from a change in personal mission. After a year or two in EMS, few people have the same personal mission as when they began.

When I first entered EMS, my highest priorities were going on good calls and being respected as a capable medic. My main interest was getting some experience under my belt, having some great stories to tell and shedding the fumbling reputation that goes with being a new guy. I had little concern about the organization, and I would have gone to work even if I had been paid half my wage.

Two years later, things were very different. My personal mission had changed: I was more interested in the professional aspects of the job, how the organization was treating me, and why the medical director was reluctant to let us do certain advanced procedures. I had changed, and it affected my relationship with the organization.

Re-examining your personal mission and taking responsibility for change can be painful. And, while it may be more comfortable to blame the organization, the rewards of being true to yourself will help you make a giant leap forward in creating success.

Taking Action

When you assess trouble with the organization, you may discover that the issue is minor and requires no action. On our canoe adventure, some trials seemed enormous. Later, with the perspective of time, my son and I found they were really just minor inconveniences. When evaluating what you want from your job, consider whether it is a battle worth fighting. If not, adjust your perspective and continue on.

Sometimes, more than perspective is needed. For ex-

> *"The only thing that is certain for man is change. To battle change is to waste one's time . . . to become the willing ally of change is to assure oneself of life."*
>
> —Leo Buscaglia

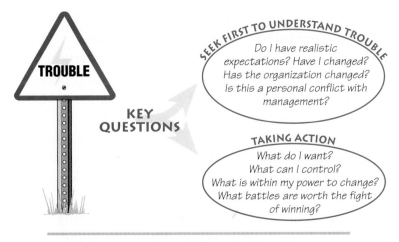

Troubleshooting in Your Relationship With Management

ample, being faithful to your personal mission may mean trying to change something in the organization. Organizations are not sacred, flawless creations; they often need changing. As a member of the organization, you have the right to suggest new ideas. Furthermore, you should work toward the things you believe. Keep in mind that changing an organization can be extremely difficult. If you are dedicated to changing something, be sure you feel strongly enough about the issue to carry it through, and then go to work on your goal. Some of the most innovative ideas in EMS come from front-line providers who carry their ideas forward and teach their managers about change. (We'll talk more about this later.)

At times, being faithful to your mission may mean leaving an organization or even pursuing a new career path; this is where many EMS people get stuck. Often, it seems easier to stay in a bad situation and complain than to move on. Granted, changing jobs or careers can be challenging and frightening, but your success may demand it. The jury is still out on whether EMS can be a lifelong career—the experts predict that most of us will change careers several times during our lives. So when you find yourself at odds

Often, it seems easier to stay in a bad situation and complain than to move on.

with the organization, ask yourself if you'd rather be doing something else.

Conflict and adversity in a relationship are not always bad. Often, they can stir things up and give birth to a whole new avenue of success. For example, one of the paramedics who was concerned about his organization's move to SSM found this seemingly negative change to be a great opportunity to learn something about himself. He had always been interested in computers and statistics, so he set out to learn the SSM software and prove to management that this

> ### *How to Propose a Change in the Organization*
>
> - **Clearly identify what needs changing.**
> - **Work out a solution and discuss it with others.**
> - **Present proposed changes in writing.**
> - **Ask for a written response.**

change was not benefiting patient care. In the process of proving his point, he discovered that he really liked computers and had a talent for working with data. He has since left street work and is working in a large computer dispatch center and consulting on the side. For this paramedic, what had appeared to be a problem became the path to a new career.

Creating a Partnership With Management

Managers and supervisors represent an organization's authority. For many EMS workers, management also represents a direct challenge to their independence. The manager is often seen as the spoiler, the police, and the mouthpiece for the higher levels of administration.

Perhaps the biggest reason EMS management has earned such a poor reputation is historical pattern. In the early days of EMS, people were promoted into management positions with no formal management training. Many of those managers employed authoritarian management styles that relied on discipline rather than tact or understanding of issues.

Fortunately, things are beginning to change. With the development of formal EMS management training programs, organizations are beginning to recognize that there is more to managing than a title and a desk. However, because of the nature of the work and the independent people EMS attracts, the relationship between management and the front line will always demand special attention.

From a front-line EMS worker's point of view, a good manager identifies with the street and understands the needs and concerns of the front line. A good manager values what medics do during the workday, including the time they are not on calls. But managers come in all shapes, sizes, abilities, and dispositions, and few will live up to the expectations of most EMS workers. Consequently, many EMS management/worker relationships suffer ongoing tension.

EMS workers often say, "I wonder what management is going to do to us next."

At the same time, managers say, "Medics want everything given to them without having to do any of the hard work."

Obviously, such attitudes do not foster teamwork or a satisfying work environment. When a manager and worker see each other as enemies, both parties' chances for success are greatly diminished.

There is a better way. While you can't change your manager, you can effect positive change in the relationship. Regardless of how good, bad, talented, or educated your manager may be, you can become more successful in the relationship by acknowledging management's role, thinking teamwork, teaching your manager well, and contributing to your manager's success.

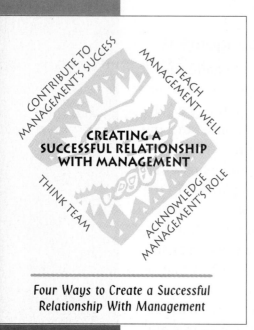

CONTRIBUTE TO MANAGEMENT'S SUCCESS

TEACH MANAGEMENT WELL

CREATING A SUCCESSFUL RELATIONSHIP WITH MANAGEMENT

THINK TEAM

ACKNOWLEDGE MANAGEMENT'S ROLE

Four Ways to Create a Successful Relationship With Management

Acknowledging Management's Role

Great calls are what make EMS exciting. No matter how long you've been in this business, the adrenaline still pumps when a big call comes in.

Yet, you couldn't go on that exciting call without a lot of important background work. You need equipment, a truck to get you there, a siren that shuts off when you turn the switch, a partner, a license for the ambulance, a medical director who will let you practice, a radio (with someone on the other end), and hopefully, a paycheck when you're all done. All of these pieces of the puzzle require management.

When confronted with poor management, you might find yourself thinking, "I could do my job a lot better if they'd quit interfering." Less management would undoubtedly make things better in some cases, but there is no way you can get along in EMS work without management's help.

Take the personalities out of management for a few moments. Think about the role. What should a manager do to enable you to do the best job possible?

Try This:

From uniforms to schedules to tires on the ambulance, make a list of things management coordinates for your work. Focus on some of the things that make the actual service you provide possible. Don't stop until you have made a list of at least ten items.

As you did this exercise, did you begin to appreciate the role management plays in your work? Regardless of how your manager performs, developing an appreciation and respect for the role will provide the foundation for the beginning of a working relationship. Now turn this

Regardless of how your manager performs, developing an appreciation and respect for the role will provide the foundation for the beginning of a working relationship.

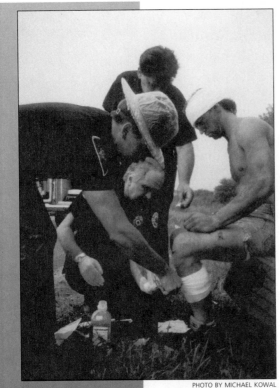

PHOTO BY MICHAEL KOWAL

idea around. Think about how nice it would be to have managers, medical directors, and the community realize the importance of what you do.

Thinking Team

I once worked for an awful manager named Jack. He had the people skills of an alligator. He communicated through short, terse notes that he left tacked up everywhere—even on the ambulance dashboard. His pet peeve was polished boots; he was convinced you couldn't run a call properly if your boots weren't mirror shiny. Jack was an easy manager to hate, but he was still an important part of the team and was vital to everyone's success.

For example, when several paramedics saw the need for a new portable radio system, Jack's support was essential to obtaining the funding. Together, Jack and the medics developed a winning proposal even though the budget was tight. When I injured my arm in a scuffle with a psychiatric patient, I needed Jack's knowledge of the incident reporting system. When several of the medics had a disagreement about who should have taken a nursing home call, Jack stepped in and made a judgment. When we considered ourselves a team and worked together, we all won. When we didn't, everyone lost.

Considering yourself and management as members of the same team may be difficult. Our culture admires lone heroes who do it all without anyone's help. But such admiration is best reserved for a good evening of Clint Eastwood movies; it will not serve your EMS work well.

Team thinking requires three acknowledgments:

1. Team thinking acknowledges that the members are stronger together than they are apart. This principle is demonstrated repeatedly in athletic teams, governments, and daily EMS work. If you respond to a serious call with one partner and no first responders, the task can become incredibly difficult. But let even a mediocre rescue service show up, and suddenly the job becomes much easier. In the same way, management is part of your team, making your performance stronger than it would be alone.

2. Team thinking acknowledges the place, role, and special abilities of each member of the team, regardless of personal bias. This principle not only applies to your partners, but to your managers as well. You don't have to like your manager to accept him as a valid member of the team. You may even believe someone else could do the job better. As a member of the team, you respect that person's special talents and abilities.

3. Team thinking acknowledges that teamwork takes practice. Perhaps nothing illustrates the value of teamwork better than multiple-casualty incidents (MCIs). Everyone in EMS has stories about disaster drills or even real disasters where everyone did their own thing and no one worked together. But EMS is finally learning how valuable practice can be. MCIs are now carefully rehearsed with all the members acting out their roles. Teamwork in the organization also takes practice. Finding a balance with your manager doesn't come automatically. You will need to try various things, see what works, and, just as in the MCI, formulate a picture of what a good relationship between management and the front line looks like.

"The team exists to accomplish a result. The community exists to support its members while they fulfill their purpose. . . . When partnerships, management teams, and organizations build communities, they tap into a greater and deeper reservoir of courage, wisdom, and productivity."

—Peter Gibb

Try This:

Reflect on how your organization would look if the front line and management began working together as a team. Try

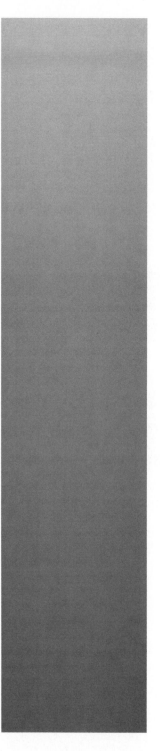

to describe what such a team would look like, assigning responsibility to all parties.

In a well-run EMS organization, management would . . .

_____

_____

_____

In a well-run EMS organization, the front line would . . .

_____

_____

_____

Thinking of management as part of the team will help eliminate the "us versus them" mentality that often characterizes EMS organizations. Working with Jack became much easier when I considered him part of the team. He never developed great management skills, but everyone learned to work around his peculiarities. As you can imagine, Jack didn't last long, and he moved on to another field of work. But another manager soon took his place. While she did not leave notes or conduct inspections, she had her own style, which added yet another dimension to the team.

Teaching Your Manager

This may come as a surprise, but one of management's main responsibilities is to serve you. You are their most important customer. The job you do on the front line is vital to the organization's success. Therefore, the manager needs you to be successful. If you handle a call well, your manager and the organization reap the benefits. The service you provide is the real product—management's job is to see that you have what you need to do your job well.

Management doesn't always know what you need. Frequently, managers who have been promoted through the ranks assume they know what EMS workers need. Often they're wrong. Most managers need you to teach them what you need to do your job well.

The word "teach" is used deliberately. First of all, teaching is very different from complaining or demanding. How you approach management with your needs will often determine the outcome.

Second, teaching is usually a planned process. Consider what it's like to teach CPR to lay people. Patiently, you talk about the theory and then demonstrate chest compressions and ventilations. As the students bend over the mannequin for the first time and attempt the skill, it's obvious they don't understand. So you calmly teach them and let them try again.

The same slow, patient process is often needed in teaching management about your needs. For example, a group of paramedics was working a set of difficult rotating shifts that continually left everyone tired and out of balance. Management began the shift rotation as a way to eliminate overtime. Of course the medics complained. At first, all management heard was the complaint, and because it was accustomed to hearing complaints, it didn't take them seriously. Nothing changed.

Most of the medics gave up. "See," they said bitterly, "management doesn't care about our needs."

But a few medics didn't let the failed first attempt stop them. They knew they could do their job more effectively—and better represent the organization—if they were well-rested and had a different schedule. They set out to teach management what it needed to know.

The medics gathered research on shift work, circadian rhythms, and sleep deprivation. They talked with their colleagues and gathered anecdotal information on specific instances in which rotating shifts had caused problems. Then they described the need in writing and made an appointment to talk with management again. This

Most managers need you to teach them what you need to do your job well.

time, management listened, but it had concerns about changing a system that was already in place. Nothing changed.

The medics were discouraged, but they didn't give up. They still believed they could do their job better if they changed the schedule. They met with their co-workers and, with management's concerns in mind, formulated several solutions that would meet the needs of both parties. Once again, they went back to management, but this time, they offered solutions. Management ultimately saw the importance of the issue and invited the medics to form a committee to work on a change.

These medics valued themselves and their work enough to go through the process of teaching management about their needs. They could have accepted management's first rejection and then spent their shifts

How to Teach Your Manager Well

1. Start by thinking of needs and solutions instead of complaints.

2. Introduce your need to management verbally in a positive manner and leave. Don't worry about the response at this time—just plant seeds.

3. After several days to several weeks, present your need again with several written solutions or options. Listen to management's response. Take note of management's concerns, especially the ones between the lines. Don't argue.

4. Considering management's response, go over your solutions again. See if you can modify them to meet management's concerns—or at least package them differently so management's concerns are met.

5. Present your need with the modified solutions to management, in writing, and request a written response.

6. Don't expect management to applaud your efforts; find your reward in the work itself. Don't quit until you have what you need to do your work well.

complaining. They could have accepted the rejection as proof that management called all the shots and had no interest in their needs. But instead, they proactively taught their managers about their need.

There are many ways to teach your manager, but the important thing to remember is that teaching is a process. Introduce the idea, support it with data, and offer solutions. Be patient with the process, and you will discover that your needs are vitally important to the organization's success.

Contributing to Your Manager's Success

Many great scientific breakthroughs occur when people turn old ideas upside down and consider an entirely new perspective. When the astronomer Copernicus hypothesized that the sun—not the earth—was the center of the universe, his views were met with skepticism. But Copernicus was right, and our understanding of the solar system took a giant leap forward. Sometimes a revolutionary idea is needed to make a big difference.

Here's a revolutionary idea for working with EMS management: Start contributing to your manager's success. This is not to suggest that you play politics or cozy up to your boss, which would draw animosity from your co-workers. Contributing to your manager's success means looking at things from his perspective. It's a step toward creating your own success.

One of management's impressions is that EMS workers are only interested in themselves and what they want. Managers often assume that the front line does not see the bigger picture. A manager's day is filled with requests and complaints—"We need to do this." "Can't you fix that?" "Where's my vacation request?"

Admittedly, listening and acting on behalf of the front line are part of a manager's job. Consider what would happen if the dynamic suddenly changed. Instead of ask-

> Contributing to your manager's success means looking at things from his perspective. It's a step toward creating your own success.

"To the degree you give others what they want, they will give you what you want!"

—Robert Conklin

ing what management was going to do for you, what if you began to contribute to your manager's success? What if you began to take action toward helping your manager be more successful? The entire nature of the relationship would change. Here's why it works.

Contributing to your manager's success dispels both parties' notion that one is serving the other. You begin to create a partnership in which you become mutual assets instead of liabilities. You begin to realize that you and your manager have many of the same goals. Furthermore, as you contribute to your manager's success, you develop a relationship that is built on respect and mutual effort toward making the work successful for both sides.

Success has a ripple effect. By contributing to your manager's success, you strengthen the entire team. There is always a bountiful fall-out from success. When a professional baseball team wins the World Series, the entire community benefits. The same is true in EMS. If your manager is successful, you and your co-workers will benefit.

A paramedic who was having a difficult time with his manager was advised to stop fighting and offer to help the manager succeed. He thought the idea was crazy, but he gave it a try. The manager didn't trust the paramedic when he began contributing to his success; he thought it was a ploy to cause trouble. Similarly, the paramedic expected to be taken advantage of. But slowly, as the worker's efforts began to have an effect on the manager's success, their relationship began to change. The men began to see each other as a part of the solution, not the problem. Together, they created a new formula for the boss/worker relationship with benefits for both sides.

How you contribute to your manager's success will be unique to your organization. Generally, managers are responsible for keeping the operation running smoothly, solving problems, and coordinating various activities. You can contribute to all of these areas.

Try This:

Consider the person to whom your immediate manager or supervisor reports. What are the criteria for your manager's success? When does the organization consider your manager or supervisor successful? Complete the follow sentence from a management perspective.

My manager is successful when . . .

_____

_____

_____

_____

Then describe how you might contribute to your manager's success. _____

_____

_____

_____

"Treat people as if they were what they ought to be, and you help them become what they are capable of being."

—Goethe

In most organizations, managers are considered to be more qualified, better educated, and more successful than the front-line workers. This is not true in EMS. There are many bright, talented, and educated people in this business who love working on the front line and don't "progress" into management. Everyone on an EMS team can benefit if they work together to help each other succeed.

Organizations and managers are not static things. Just when you think you've got them figured out, they change, but change need not affect you negatively. Your success in EMS depends much more on you than on the organization or the manager. Learning early to work with both will smooth the way toward finding the favorable outcome you want from this work.

Summary

✔ Developing a satisfying relationship with the organization and management can be difficult in EMS.

✔ How you view the organization, as good or evil, is important. In most cases, it's neither.

✔ Understand what really makes your organization tick. What is its real mission?

✔ Bridge the gap between what the organization wants and what you want.

✔ Create a partnership with management by

1) Acknowledging management's necessary role

2) Thinking of your relationship in terms of a team

3) Teaching your manager about your needs

Suggested Reading

The Addictive Organization, by Anne Wilson-Schaef and Diane Fassel (Harper & Row, San Francisco, 1988). Anne Wilson-Schaef and Diane Fassel make an excellent presentation on why some people give so much to an organization and yet come away feeling used, off-balance, and uneasy about the relationship. There is a lot of dysfunction in EMS organizations, and this book can be useful in sorting it out.

EMS Management: Beyond the Street, 2nd ed., by Joseph J. Fitch (Jems Communications, Carlsbad, California, 1993). This is the standard textbook of everything you ever wanted to know about EMS management. Although it is dry reading, it is the only comprehensive guide out there. If you want to understand management or join management, this book must be on your shelf.

Principle Centered Leadership, by Stephen R. Covey (Summit Books, New York, 1991). Stephen Covey is the Socrates of doing the right thing. This book is for anyone who aspires to be a leader. Most people in EMS will be leaders in one way or another; this book will assist you in doing it right. Covey also gives a good picture of what a balanced principled leader should be like.

You Don't Have to Go Home from Work Exhausted, by Ann McGee-Cooper (Bowen & Rogers, Dallas, 1990). This is a great guide to learning how to have more fun with your work. It will teach you how to relax and have more energy in the midst of a busy life. The illustrations alone are worth the price.

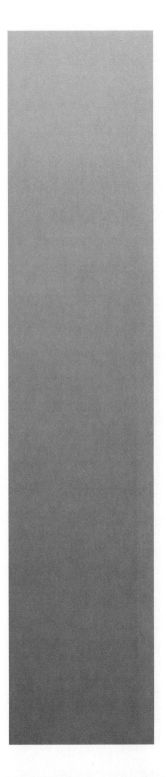

8 | Creating Community

Men come together to keep alive; they stay together to live a good life.

—Aristotle

In the popular action movie *Die Hard*, Bruce Willis plays an out-of-town cop named John McClain, who confronts a group of hardened terrorists who have taken over an office building. Hostages are being held, including McClain's wife, and he alone—tired, barefoot, and armed only with his service revolver—must save the day.

The lone hero fighting for victory against hordes of bad guys is a popular theme in our society, one that is deeply rooted in our culture. We glorify the individual and his ability to make it on his own. We admire the person who takes the less popular path. We honor those who distinguish themselves from the rest of society. We champion the attributes of rugged individualism, savor the freedom of "being ourselves," and shudder at the idea of being just one of the crowd.

This notion of the heroic individual is very prevalent in EMS. Who hasn't dreamed of finding himself alone in a heroic situation where skills and abilities are desperately needed to save a life? Of course, it's not that we seek glory; we just want to help. It's our duty to step in, perhaps reluctantly, and save the day. If someone was to make an EMS action movie, it would certainly feature a barefoot EMT or paramedic, caught alone in the middle of a dramatic disaster with little equipment and certainly no medical direction. The ending? You guessed it: By sheer MacGyveresque ability and a *Die Hard* determination, the lone EMS worker would be victorious.

The heroic loner theme is a myth. It's just a story. In history and in real life, there are no such creatures. No matter how romantic it sounds, you cannot make it on your own. Even the *Die Hard* hero doesn't really do it alone. As the story unfolds, the hero becomes aware of his limitations, his fear of failure, and the foolishness of his oversized ego. He needs help, if nothing more than the encouragement to keep going and the knowledge that he is not alone. Help

"Community is like pornography, to paraphrase Justice Brennan: I don't know how to define it, but I sure as hell know it when I see it."

—A federal judge attending a community building workshop

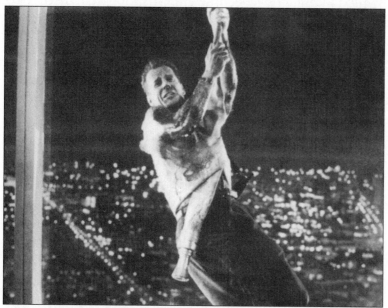

© PETER SOREL, 1988 20TH CENTURY FOX/MOTION PICTURE AND TELEVISION PHOTO ARCHIVE

Bruce Willis plays lone cop John McClain in the movie Die Hard. *Even in the movie, the "lone hero" story is a myth.*

"One of the things a community is not, is a simple geographical aggregate of people."

—M. Scott Peck

comes from a local cop who talks with McClain on a police radio. There is great contrast between the two characters. McClain is the hard-boiled hero, his helper a washed-up street cop who doubts his own ability. Yet, as they begin talking to each other on the radio, something powerful happens. They become a "community."

What Is Community?

The word "community" may make you think of many things. Community can refer to where you live. It can also refer to a group of people, such as the medical community, the African-American community, the business community, the scientific community, the gay community, or even the EMS community. These descriptive uses of the word help us talk about a group as one entity. But there is a concept of community that is more than just a description.

When the *Die Hard* hero and the self-doubting cop begin talking, they become much more than their two abilities added together. Describing exactly what they become is difficult, because true community is such a large, intangible concept. It's like trying to describe electricity. You can't deny the reality of electricity. It keeps your clock radio running all night and wakes you up in the morning. It lights the bathroom as you brush your teeth, and it turns over your car's engine. There's no doubting electricity's power, but even an electrical engineer would be at a loss to explain it comprehensively. True community is the same—difficult to describe, mysterious, but undeniable when it happens.

In the late '70s, I was a founding member of a small hospital-based ALS service on the western edge of the Twin Cities. The odds of the service becoming anything of substance were slim. There was strong local support for the old volunteer ambulance service, and the medical community was skeptical that ALS was necessary. In addition, the service area was bordered by several large, well-funded ALS services, which attracted most of the good talent.

In spite of the odds, a small group of paramedics, EMTs, and doctors came together and accomplished something extraordinary. The group became more than just the sum of its parts—it became a community full of vitality and power. Everyone who participated was aware that something special was happening. Together, the group struggled, dreamed, cried, worked, fought, and ultimately achieved something great. Through numerous setbacks, difficult handicaps, and a frustrating administration, the group created a dynamic service that has become a leader in its area in terms of quality, advanced skills, and a rewarding work environment.

Many of the original founders have left, but every few years the group gets together to reminisce about old times. They don't focus on the big EMS achievements. Instead, people talk about the rewards and satisfaction that came from working together and creating this mysterious thing called community.

Several years ago, I surveyed several hundred EMS workers from throughout the United States about what they would miss most if they left EMS. Few mentioned the big, dramatic calls or the last-minute saves. Almost to a person, they said they'd miss community the most. In creating success in EMS, one of the most enduring and satisfying parts of this work is not the excitement of saving a life, but the community we create with others. The romantic idea of the heroic loner doesn't work in EMS because you need other people. You need others not just to lift the stretcher and apply a backboard, but for a mutual creation of success.

Spontaneous Communities and Created Communities

Communities like the one created in *Die Hard* are

> One of the most enduring and satisfying parts of this work is not the excitement of saving a life, but the community we create with others.

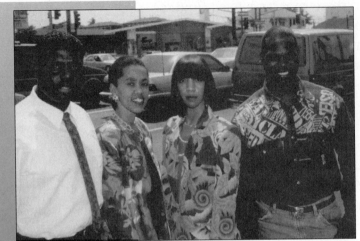

The "Heroes in the Hood" (l-r) were Titus Murphy, Lei Yuille, Terri Barnett, and Bobby Green. These four strangers created a community and saved truck driver Reginald Denny during the 1992 Los Angeles riots.

PHOTO BY JOHN BARR/LIAISON INTERNATIONAL

spontaneous occurrences driven by a crisis or a specific, temporary need. The community exists for the life of the crisis and often disappears when the need goes away. Despite their temporary nature, spontaneous communities are great models for learning how to create communities in your everyday work and life.

During the dark, violent hours of the South Central Los Angeles riots in 1992, there were many examples of spontaneous community. While the media focused on rioters, looters, and arsonists, many people joined together to help the injured, put out fires, and protect property. One highly reported example of spontaneous community occurred at the corner of Normandie and Florence where four people risked their lives to aid truck driver Reginald Denny. Denny was driving a large gravel truck when he was stopped by an angry mob. He was dragged from his truck, robbed, beaten with bricks, hit with a hammer, kicked repeatedly, and shot at with a shotgun. The entire brutal incident was reported live by an overhead news helicopter.

Four people were stirred to action and raced to help. As Denny—dazed, confused, and bleeding—managed to crawl back into his truck and attempted to drive away, Lei Yuille jumped onto the truck's passenger side running board and began directing him to a nearby restaurant.

As the truck inched forward, Titus Murphy and Terri

Barnett broke through the rioting crowd and jumped onto the driver side running board to help. Murphy immediately realized Denny could not drive and that he was rapidly losing consciousness. Then Bobby Green, also a truck driver, arrived. He had seen the beating on television and had come to help a fellow truck driver. Green moved into the driver's seat.

Without discussion, the four people spontaneously helped take Denny to a hospital—no easy task in the riot-filled streets. Moments earlier they had been strangers; now they were a community.

Barnett jumped into her blue Honda Civic to lead the procession. Murphy remained on the running board so he could shout directions to Green, who could barely see through the smashed windshield. Yuille moved to the passenger seat to comfort Denny, who had a large laceration on his face and was covered with blood. Honking their way through traffic, the group made its way to the hospital. Just as they arrived, Denny began to seize. He was immediately rushed into emergency surgery, where two blood clots were removed from his brain. A hospital spokesperson later said Denny would not have survived if he had arrived at the hospital any later.

This story of people working together in a crisis is not new to EMS workers. It happens every day in medical emergencies. What makes these spontaneous communities work? How is it that total strangers can come together and, regardless of who they are or what they represent, accomplish something together they could not do alone? Three important elements make a spontaneous community work.

First, the need for community is recognized. Helping Reginald Denny in the midst of a riot was not a job for a lone hero. Every helpful hand was critical. No one could do what needed to be done alone. The four rescuers instinctively recognized that they needed each other.

"We were the first ones on the scene—the only uniformed rescuers. At first we were overwhelmed. It was more than we could handle alone. Suddenly these people started coming up. Guys in baseball caps, guys in suits, a woman with several blankets. With all the blood and the fear of AIDS these days, you don't expect people to help, but there was a whole group of people trying to help us get those kids out of there."

—An EMT describing an accident involving a van full of school children

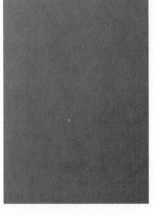

"Synergy is everywhere in nature. If you plant two plants close together, the roots commingle and improve the quality of the soil so that both plants grow better than if they were separated. If you put two pieces of wood together, they will hold much more than the total of the weight held by each separately. The whole is greater than the sum of its parts. One plus one equals three or more."

—Stephen R. Covey

The second ingredient is a natural respect for one another. It didn't matter that Los Angeles was being torn apart around them; the rescuers respected each other's abilities to help. Green didn't need to produce his truck driver's license. No one questioned Murphy's ability to navigate. No one worried whether Barnett could lead the procession or handle the sight of blood. Everyone respected one other as human beings with something to offer the situation.

The third element of spontaneous communities is that everyone focuses on a vital common purpose. Getting Reginald Denny to the hospital became the rescuers' shared goal. They were not thinking about what they could gain from the experience, how they could win or lose, or how their feat would play in the news. The possibility that they could even be killed for involving themselves didn't stop them. Together, they focused on a common purpose.

All three of these elements may appear so obvious in a crisis situation that they seem foolish to discuss. But what about when there is no crisis? How do you create community in your EMS work apart from what occurs spontaneously? Community is created by consciously recognizing the need for community, acting with respect, and focusing on something bigger than yourself. Let's take a closer look at each of these elements.

Recognizing the Need for Community

When running a cardiac arrest, your need for others is obvious. You need someone to perform CPR, a partner to start an IV, and someone to manage the airway. You need others to get a backboard, comfort the family, and hold the door when you head for the ambulance. What about when the cardiac arrest is over and you are back at the station? Do you still need others?

Many paramedics and EMTs don't believe they need community beyond the emergency scene. The evidence

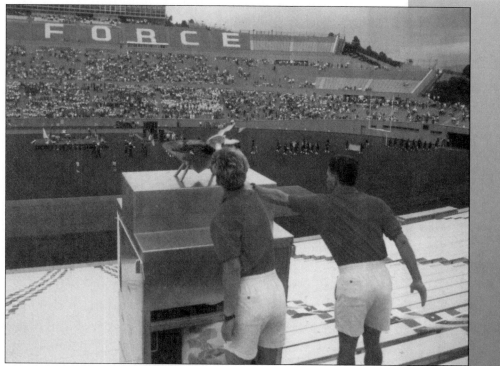

PHOTO BY JIM MALLORY/CONSULTING SYSTEMS, INC.

Thousands of first responders from all over the world participated in the 1993 World Fire and Police Games in Colorado Springs, Colorado. Competitors create a community outside of emergency service.

for this is seen in the lack of a strong, collective EMS workers' voice in shaping the industry. Many complain about "what's done to us" by the industry, management, and the medical community. Yet, few join associations, form action groups, or work with others to shape their future. They don't recognize their need for one another and the strength of community outside of emergency situations.

This blindness to the need for community may account for the difficulty some EMS workers have working with each other. Many paramedics request tools for getting along with "difficult" co-workers.

"I need something that will help me get along with Bill," one paramedic said. "I work with this guy three times a week and just dread it. He's such a jerk, I just wish he'd go do something else for a living. Nothing works with Bill."

The complaining paramedic did not see the value of community. He didn't have any need for Bill apart from the calls they did together. All the interpersonal skills in the world could not help him get along with others if he didn't first see a need.

When you first realize you need others, you will begin to find ways to get along. There is an old story about a man lost in the woods who wanders about taking different paths and directions. No matter what he tries, he never finds his way. Then one day, in the midst of great discouragement, he sees another man coming through the trees. His spirits soar. "I've been found," he says.

He runs toward the man, happily shouting his relief. As he approaches, however, he discovers that the other man is lost, too. His shoulders slump with disappointment.

This is how we often feel about co-workers in EMS; apart from the calls, we don't need them. They're in the same boat as we are, so what could we possibly gain from them? They're just as lost or unhappy as we are. We might as well go on our separate ways.

As the two lost men turn to go their separate ways, one suddenly recognizes the benefit of community.

"Hey, I've got an idea," he says excitedly. "Sure we're both lost, but if you show me where you've been and I show you where I've been, we won't have to cover the same ground. We'll combine our experience and improve our chances of finding our way out." They do what he suggests, and they leave the woods together.

The lost men grasped the most important element of community: their need for each other.

In looking deeper into this story, we find that the lost men find more than just a path out of the woods. They talk, and they discover that they come from very

> **When you first realize you need others, you will begin to find ways to get along.**

different backgrounds, but have something to offer each other. Together, they reduce the monotony of walking by sharing stories and jokes. Together, they battle the discouragement of being lost. When several bears threaten them, they make such a commotion together that the bears run away.

During their travels, one of the men criticizes himself for having become lost in the first place. The other man points out that even the best hikers occasionally lose their way.

The men do not always agree. They often have loud, passionate disagreements about where to sleep and which path to take. But they work it out because they realize that together they are much stronger than they were apart.

The men remain friends. Through the years, they often visit each other and reminisce about their ordeal. Whenever either of them has a crisis, the other shows up to do what he can. Together, they are stronger than they would be on their own.

The first element of creating community is the belief that you need other people and the recognition that with others, you are more. If you're not convinced you need community, it can't be created. You'll enjoy the spontaneous communities of emergencies, but you won't have a community in everyday life. You'll gravitate toward the people you like and those who like you, and there will be some good times, but you will not create community.

The lost men gained more than a safe escape from the woods. Likewise, you need others in EMS for more than the calls. If you are to be successful in this career, you need people you can laugh and cry with—people to help you over the rough spots. You need people who can tell you you're wrong and people who can encourage you to do what's right. Your co-workers need the same from you. Together, your accomplishments as a community will far exceed what you might do on your own.

> The community's accomplishments will far exceed what you might do on your own.

Managing Differences

What is the best way for people to manage differences? Roger Fisher and William Ury of the Harvard Negotiation Project and authors of *Getting to Yes* point out that we often try to solve differences by bargaining over our positions. We wind up seeing solutions where one or the other party wins or no one wins, but not where both parties win. They suggest negotiating for solutions where both parties win by

- Separating people from the problem
- Focusing on interests instead of positions
- Seeking and, if necessary, inventing options for mutual gain
- Negotiating a settlement from objective criteria and principles

Acting With Respect

When working with others, we often approach getting along in terms of liking others and being liked. This is only natural. The most envied kids in school were the ones everyone liked, and the popular people in your organization are the "likable" ones. Thus, you might be compelled to try to create your community by being liked and by liking others. But community is actually built through mutual respect.

To respect someone means moving beyond the emotion of liking or disliking that person and beginning to value his unique attributes, talents, and abilities. Respect is about recognizing another person's ability to contribute to the community in his own unique way. This raises an important question: How do you respect someone if you don't particularly like that person?

In his fascinating book on community titled *The Different Drum*, M. Scott Peck tells a wonderful story about a monastery that sounds like many EMS communities. The old monastery had fallen on hard times. No one wanted to join because the monks were continually bickering and

Respect is about recognizing another person's ability to contribute to the community in his own unique way.

fighting among themselves. The monks were not happy—even the most simple tasks had become laborious because no one worked together.

The head of the monastery, a thoughtful old abbot, was very concerned. He loved the monks but couldn't figure out how to pull them together. He announced that he would seek the advice of a wise rabbi who often prayed alone in a small, tumbled-down shack near the monastery. When the abbot arrived at the rabbi's shack, he was greeted warmly and invited in. He sank wearily into a chair and began sharing his problems. The rabbi listened intently. When the abbot finished, the rabbi shook his head and pulled thoughtfully at his long beard.

"Ahhh, it's terrible. Terrible," he said. "But I don't know what to tell you." They sat in silence for a long while, and finally the abbot got up to leave. He hadn't really expected an easy answer, and he appreciated the rabbi's listening. Just as he was going out the door, the rabbi said, "Oh yes, there is one thing I can tell you. The messiah is among you."

When the abbot got back to the monastery, the monks gathered around and asked what the rabbi had said. The abbot told them that unfortunately, the rabbi didn't know what to do either. Then he told them, "As I was leaving, the rabbi said, 'The messiah is among you.' I don't know what he meant. It must be some old cryptic saying." The monks agreed that it was nothing and returned to their duties. As they worked, they began to think about what the rabbi had said. "What if the messiah is really among us?" they wondered. Slowly, they began to ponder the virtues and quirks of their brethren. It couldn't be crabby old Philip, they said, but he does have a way with animals. It couldn't be arrogant Andrew, but he does know how to organize things. Eventually, each monk even considered himself. The rabbi couldn't have meant me, each thought, although I do

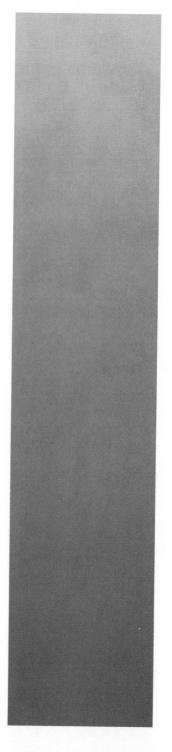

have a way with the scriptures . . . or I do feel close to those who suffer.

As the monks continued to consider the possibilities, they began to change. Slowly, they began to recognize the value of each other and the value of themselves. Even though they were very different people, they began to respect their differences. That respect continued to grow. Soon they were once again a community others wanted to join.

In pursuing the myth of the lone hero, many EMS workers become like the monks. They fail to value themselves and their co-workers and therefore have no basis for common respect. Every human being is endowed with special gifts, abilities, and attributes. Respect grows from an appreciation of an individual's uniqueness. When people begin to act with respect toward each other, they move beyond an emotional reaction, and community begins to build.

Try This:

Make a list of the people with whom you work most closely. Without thinking about whether you like each person, write something you respect about him or her.

_____

_____

_____

_____

_____

_____

Focusing on a Vital Common Purpose

When people spontaneously form communities during a crisis, they respond to a common need that is bigger than their individual needs. When creating everyday

Life Link III provides critical care ground and air transport.

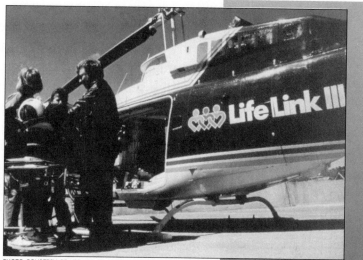

PHOTO COURTESY OF LIFE LINK III

communities, the members must share a vital common purpose. As pointed out in Chapter Three, purpose is not something you manufacture. Purpose is discovered. Stop and ask yourself what unites you and your co-workers. What concerns do you share? What are your common dreams, desires, and aspirations? What common obstacles are you trying to overcome?

One of the most exciting EMS communities that I know of exists among workers at Life Link III, a nonprofit, critical care ground and air transport service in St. Paul, Minnesota. These workers, many of whom have worked at Life Link for years, have a powerful common interest in EMS that challenges the limits of medical transportation. This interest has become a vital uniting force that has spawned a potent and extremely close community.

It's exciting to be around this community of mavericks. They are always talking about doing things better, tapping each other's talents, and inventing and modifying equipment. One afternoon, they received a call from a South Dakota Indian reservation where a new mother and her critically ill twins needed transportation to a large medical center. The situation required two aircraft, extensive neonatal equipment, personnel, and unique teamwork. The team raced to action. Everyone worked together, and in no time the planes were off the ground and on the way to yet another unusual transport. What energizes and drives this community is a vital common purpose.

What energizes and drives community is a vital common purpose.

"Communities are places or entities where each member can give something, where each can contribute something that he feels especially able to give, something that he is good at. The gift from each member is valued by the whole community, and all the gifts are unique. The gift that the community gives back to each member is that of a role and a connection."

—Ed Margason

A community's purpose need not be lofty and altruistic. For ten years, I have been part of a unique community of twelve EMS and former EMS people called the Winders. The group gets together several times throughout the year to ski, golf, or just spend several days together away from EMS work. The group formed out of a common need to unwind from the everyday pressures of EMS and to be with people who understood the ups and downs of street work. In the beginning, it just seemed like a lot of fun. No one was thinking about community, yet because there is a common vital purpose, the Winders have become a powerful community that goes beyond just having fun. There is now a special bond between members. For better or worse, we can always count on being accepted, helped, and encouraged by each other. No one imagined it would last this long; then again, none of us was familiar with the power of community.

Often, a common adversary can bring about community. One group of paramedics had a common adversary in the management of their organization. The organization consistently took advantage of them, requiring overtime and mandatory "holdovers,"—all with substandard pay. The paramedics were drawn together because they had a common problem.

History books are full of communities brought together by a common enemy. This may be the genesis of your community. The danger with such communities is that when the enemy ceases to be a threat, the community may fall apart.

You don't need an adversary to begin creating community. You can begin by simply considering the common interests you share with your co-workers. Those interests can be as ordinary as a desire for work that is challenging and rewarding.

Such a desire goes hand-in-hand with creating community. One of the most rewarding aspects of EMS work may be the relationships you cultivate with others. People can endure all kinds of difficulties, hardships, and disappointments in life if they have a strong community to support them. You must create your own success, but one of your greatest successes in EMS work could be the community you create.

Storytelling—the Fabric of Community

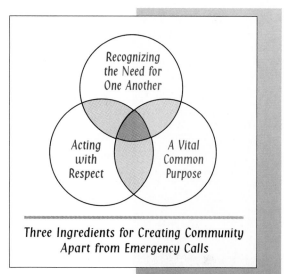

Three Ingredients for Creating Community Apart from Emergency Calls

Imagine the end of a difficult shift. You've had several intense calls and are preparing to go home. The new crew comes in and asks about your shift. You mention your calls, and then, for some unexplained reason, you begin to elaborate on one of the calls. It was an old farmer who had had a heart attack in his barn. You set the scene, mentioning the frantic wife, the smell of hay and manure, and the look on the man's face. You continue beyond the mere medical explanation, talking about how you felt, what the farmer said to you, and how uncertain you were as you watched the PVCs dance across your monitor.

The new crew has stopped checking out the rig. They listen with eyes wide as you gesture and recreate the moment when the old farm dog came to nuzzle his master and say good-bye. The new crew asks a few questions and compliments your performance. One of the crew members begins to tell about a similar call he once had. His voice changes as he launches into the tale, and you settle back to listen. When he finishes, your partner tells about another call. You've heard this story at least a half dozen times before, but it doesn't matter; it's part of the ritual. More stories are told, and you finally realize it's long past quitting time.

One of your greatest successes in EMS work could be the community you create.

Storytelling is the fabric of EMS communities. Stories are the oral history of your accomplishments and common interests. Stories are the EMS community's mythology. Storytelling is a powerful ritual that draws people together.

The three elements of community are all realized when stories are told. The entire setting of storytelling, with long-winded tellers and willing listeners, is an acknowledgment of the need for community. More than that, through hearing and telling stories, people open up and reveal parts of themselves in such a way that new value and respect are discovered. Furthermore, as stories are told, common interests of the group are found. Storytelling is indeed a powerful tool for building community.

Unfortunately, EMS people often shy away from telling stories from the heart. Everyone has run into that one war story instructor who is always telling disgusting tales of blood and guts. No one wants to get the reputation of telling too many war stories. Thus, stories are often told in cryptic medical and technological terms. "We had a C-arrest. The guy was in refractory V-fib and we couldn't get the tube, learned he was a DNR, so we DC'ed everything and cleared." Such reporting diminishes the many dimensions of your work. It ignores that there is much more to a call than the medical aspects. There are colors, smells, sounds, and people other than the patient. On every call, there are feelings and observations that are as much a part of the experience as the actual patient care.

What happens when you tell a story or listen to one told by a co-worker? By its very nature, storytelling becomes a community activity. Watch what happens when a group of EMS people begin to swap tales. People move in closer. Everyone participates by listening or telling. In storytelling, walls are lowered, guards are dropped, and vulnerabilities are revealed. You can't tell a story without giving glimpses of your true self.

Stories are the EMS community's mythology.

I once witnessed the powerful community aspect of storytelling. After a call, a group of EMS people and firefighters began swapping tales about motorcycle wrecks. At first they laughed about helmetless riders, Harleys, and motorcycle girls. Then one person told a story of a cyclist who had hit a train at an unmarked crossing in the middle of the night. Another told the story of a "crotch rocket" sailing over a fence and into a river. One of the older firefighters softly mentioned that his only daughter had been killed on a motorcycle.

Suddenly the room grew quiet, and everyone moved closer. As the man fidgeted with an unlit cigarette, he revealed something about himself no one had known before. Years earlier, on a beautiful summer day, his daughter had hopped onto the back of a neighbor's motor scooter against her father's wishes. She died moments later in front of his house when the scooter slid into a passing truck. The man's eyes filled with tears as he told the story. As he tried to turn away, a fellow firefighter clamped his arm around the man's shoulder and pulled him close. His vulnerability had a powerful effect on the group, and for several hours people leaned against the fire trucks and talked.

When we tell stories, not only do we learn about each other, we also give the community a chance to help us heal our wounds. And is this not what a community should really be about? Formal critical incident stress debriefing sessions (discussed in Chapter Nine) demonstrate the vital importance of talking about our calls with each other. When a story is told, the teller not only relays the events, but he gets in touch with the emotional side of this work.

Many times, I have not realized the magnitude of a call until I begin to tell it. More than once, my voice has cracked in the middle of a tale, and I suddenly become aware of my emotions. We find release in telling a story. It's almost as if by telling the story, we let it go. Such storytelling and honest healing can only happen in a community of people who understand the work, the triumphs, and the hurts.

Beyond healing, storytelling is a powerful communal celebration of what EMS is all about. Heroic work has always been honored in storytelling; for thousands of years, people have told the tales of heroic deeds as a means of celebrating what's accomplished. EMS is much more than fast medical technology on wheels. From the dispatcher's initial page to the sights and sounds of the scene to the feelings in the gut—all are part of this work. Only in storytelling can such things be celebrated.

One of the best ways you can begin to see the power of community is by telling stories. Look for those spontaneous moments when stories are being told. Listen and then tell a few of your own. Watch what happens.

Try This:

Make a list of stories you would like to tell. Think back over your work in EMS and make a list of your interesting experiences. Include the big, four-alarm calls, as well as the humorous, ordinary, or touching experiences. Make your list by giving each story a descriptive name such as:

- *Arrest at the church communion altar*
- *Old lady with thirty cats*
- *The Halloween prank*
- *Double fatal on Highway 7*
- *The exploding mast suit*
- *He took two stretchers*

Have fun, and make your list as long as you like. You'll discover you have more stories than you suspected.

In making this list, you have planted a seed in your subconscious that will remind you of each story at an appropriate time.

Where to Start

Unlike spontaneous communities, the community you create among your fellow EMS workers will not happen all at once. It will take an investment of time. It may be the best investment you make in your EMS work.

You can begin by treating your co-workers with respect. Assume that they deserve your respect and let that assumption guide your actions. Put aside your judgments and begin to tune into what you have in common rather than how you are different. Such actions begin to plant seeds of trust. As those seeds grow, you will build the framework of community.

Don't make the mistake of holding too tightly to the myth of the lone hero. In *Die Hard*, when it appears as if the lone hero has rescued everyone and saved the day, McClain suddenly finds himself in desperate need of help. A terrorist has leveled a gun at him and is about to kill him. There is nothing he can do.

If he were on his own, it would be all over. Yet, through the power of their community, something has happened to Powell, McClain's washed-up cop buddy on the radio. Powell has changed. In the beginning, he was a frightened, broken man. Now, without hesitation, he throws his shoulders back, and shoots the terrorist. He puts to rest the notion that he or McClain can get by without community.

"If you think you can't change the world by yourself, join some people who agree."

—The motto of Business Partnership for Peace

Summary

✔ The lone hero is not a valid approach to EMS work; you need others to be successful.

✔ One of the most satisfying aspects of EMS comes from the community EMS people form together.

✔ Spontaneous communities created in crisis are

good models for creating planned communities apart from crisis.

✔ The need for community must be recognized.

✔ Actions toward others must be founded in respect.

✔ Community emerges out of a vital common purpose.

✔ Storytelling is often the fabric of community life.

Suggested Reading

Creating Community Anywhere, by Carolyn R. Shaffer and Kristin Anundsen (Jeremy P. Tarcher/Perigee, New York, 1993). This unique book shows why we need community in our day and culture. Included is a starter kit on how to build your own community.

The Different Drum: Community-Making and Peace, by M. Scott Peck, M.D. (Simon and Schuster, New York, 1987). If the idea of community interests you, this is the book for you. Dr. Peck is a psychiatrist who shows why it is so important to make the leap from individual growth to community growth and why we all need each other.

EMT: Rescue, by Pat Ivy (Ivy Books, New York, 1993). Pat Ivy's second book on being an EMT provides a compelling look at an EMS community. The EMS experiences described show how important a close community is to success in EMS. This is a good all-around read and well worth the five dollars.

Getting to Yes: Negotiating Agreement Without Giving In, by Roger Fisher and William Ury with Bruce Patton (Penguin Books, New York, 1981). The secret to working cooperatively with others is learning to handle disagreements in such a way that both parties win. This is a short guide to handling the negotiations we carry on in everyday life. This book should be required reading for anyone who has to work with a partner in crisis situations.

Rescue Alert, by Joan E. Lloyd and Edwin B. Herman (Berkley Books, New York, 1994). Here is another book about an EMS community—the Fairfax Volunteer Ambulance Corps. Of course, the main focus of the book is on the rescues, but you'll notice the importance of the community between the lines. A sense of community is what makes these organizations work so well.

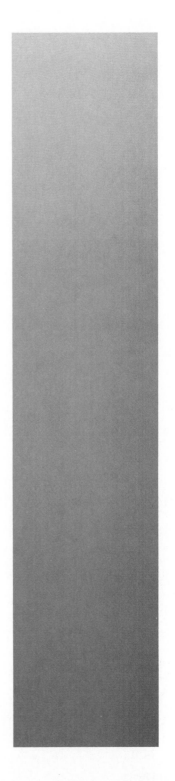

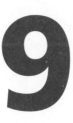

9 Opportunities in Tough Stuff

The deeper sorrow carves into your being, the more joy you can contain.

—Kahlil Gibran

It's afternoon, and the shift has been slow. Earlier that day, you were called to a nursing home to pick up a confused elderly lady with a high temperature. Your partner attended. Now it's your turn.

While waiting for the next call, you read a letter from your sister. She is bragging about your favorite niece and how well she's doing in school. You smile, thinking about her sparkling brown eyes and how she bosses everyone around. Then the pager sounds.

"One down at Jefferson Elementary," the dispatcher rattles off. "Code 3." You never run to the ambulance, but something in your gut tells you this call is urgent. Your partner feels it, too, and has the engine running as you climb in. Trying to act nonchalant over the sound of the siren, your partner says, "Probably just a seizure."

But as you near the school, a police officer's voice comes across the radio. He's out of breath, and he's talking in short gasps. He says to use the auditorium entrance and pleads for you to hurry. Without slowing, your partner swings into the school driveway and drives past several yellow buses. You grab a drug box and race into the auditorium. It's dark, but your eyes quickly adjust. Several people are bent over a small figure on the brightly lit stage.

Vaulting onto the stage, you drop to your knees beside her. She is 8 or 9 years old, a small child dressed in a bright pink leotard, white tights, and delicate ballet slippers. Her neck is arched back in an unnatural stretch, and there is a tight, almost imperceptible jerking in her arms and hands. A frantic gray-haired woman is trying to wipe vomit away from the girl's clenched mouth. One of the adults tells you the girl was dancing when she suddenly collapsed to the floor and started shaking. You quickly clear the airway and begin a survey. Her whole body is rigid. Her eyes are blank and are twitching to one side. Her respirations are shallow, fast, and noisy. You realize this is no ordinary seizure.

As your partner looks for an IV on the thin arm, you feel hollow in the pit of your stomach. The thrill you normally have on a good call is gone. But the professional in you focuses on airway, oxygen, IV, medical control, Valium, suction, backboard, and stretcher. Everything is being done right, but somehow, in the midst of all the action, your human side doesn't stop thinking, seeing, and feeling. Chipped red polish dots her little fingernails. Beyond the clenched jaw, the face is innocent and charming. Several other girls in ballet outfits stand near the door crying as you wheel their friend to the ambulance.

En route to the hospital, the girl becomes less rigid. The shaking stops. You let out your breath, begin to relax, and pick up the radio to give a report. Suddenly you notice that her chest is not moving. The report breaks off midsentence, and you snatch off the oxygen mask, lowering your ear to her mouth. There is nothing. You place your hand on her chest. Still nothing. A split second of

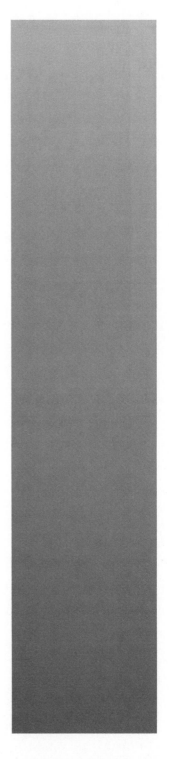

Tough Stuff—that which defies neat medical, social, and intellectual explanations—the part left out of television emergency shows.

panic hits, but just as quickly, the professional returns. By the time you reach the emergency department, you've intubated your patient and are bagging her rapidly. The little body has gone completely flaccid, and the eyes are vacant, with big, unmoving pupils.

Things do not improve in the ED. Activity swirls about the girl, but nothing works. Her pulse rate begins to drop, and before she's even off your stretcher, you are doing CPR. You can't believe how little pressure it takes to push on her small chest. Then it all comes to a quiet end as the doctor says in a flat voice, "I don't think we can do any more. Let's quit." The ending doesn't fit all of the work you've just done. There's no explanation, no celebration. Just silence. An hour ago, the little girl was dancing.

Filling out your EMS form, you feel hollow and empty. You wish you could have done more or at least know what went wrong. The doctor mentions cerebral hemorrhage and autopsy, but you need more than a medical answer.

Later, while cleaning up the ambulance at the end of your shift, you find a small, wrinkled ballet slipper wedged between the squad bench and wall. You pick it up and slowly turn it over. You find yourself thinking about your beautiful niece. This is tough stuff.

Understanding Tough Stuff

Tough stuff is the experience of human tragedy, suffering, and death in EMS. It is mysterious, uncomfortable, and often confusing. It cannot be explained with medicine and science. It may be a suicide, a rape, a runaway heart, an undramatic death in a nursing home, or a bloody, multiple-victim highway accident. Tough stuff is the part of the work for which training and practice cannot prepare you. It must be experienced.

The tough stuff is what makes EMS such a unique field of work.

The tough stuff is what makes EMS such a unique field of work. EMS deals with a segment of human life most people will not approach. We live in a culture that is largely uncomfortable with suffering and death. Since the development of modern medicine, people have increasingly left the care of the seriously ill, injured, and dying to professionals. With the industrial revolution, the urbanization of our society, and the fragmentation of extended families, caring for the dying—and death itself—moved out of the home and into the purview of "professionals."

Dr. Robert Fulton, a sociologist who studies death at the University of Minnesota, says these changes in our society have insulated most people from having contact with death. His studies show that because most deaths occur in hospitals or other institutions, people in our society have only a five percent chance of physically encountering a death in their immediate family or circle of friends before the age of 21. Consequently, people grow up gaining little experience in dealing with death and suffering, and they want to keep it that way.

When people hear that you work in EMS, they may wrinkle their noses and say, "I don't know how you can do emergency work. I couldn't handle it." And they're right. Most people can't imagine facing the tough stuff you experience every day.

Even within the medical field, EMS is unique. Other branches of medicine are practiced in the sterile, controlled environment of the hospital or clinic. You find and treat your patients in the raw, natural setting of everyday life. You find them in the elementary school, in bed, on the toilet, and under wrecked cars. The deaths you see are not neat, gentle hospice passings, but are often sudden, messy, and undignified. You do not have the protective setting of the institution. You find human suffering in the ordinary places.

Despite its everyday occurrence, tough stuff never becomes ordinary. It's not the sort of thing you can put aside when you take off your uniform. The memories remain, and like a soldier who has been to war, you are

As a medic, you do not have the protective setting of the institution. You find human suffering in the ordinary places.

affected. The question is, *how* are you affected? Tough stuff can be dangerous, but it can also present a great opportunity.

The Danger of Stress

In April 1991, EMTs in the small town of Webster, Wisconsin, responded to a call for shots being fired. A mentally unbalanced man had shot two police officers in the middle of a street near an elementary school. Before the man could escape, other police officers shot him.

When the EMTs arrived on scene, they found three victims in cardiac arrest. Some of the EMTs knew the victims personally. After a quick assessment, they began working on one of the police officers, the only victim who appeared viable. He was transported with CPR in progress to a hospital and was then flown to a large medical center.

Miraculously, the police officer survived—the EMTs had done a great job. They had performed as they were trained, but it was a bitter success. The two other men were dead, and the surviving police officer was left a quadriplegic. The EMTs could not help but wonder: Had they done everything possible? Should they have worked on the other officer? Why did this happen? In addition to the questions they asked themselves, they had to deal with an entire community's relentless questioning.

The incident caused the responders a great deal of stress. The most obvious danger of tough stuff is the psychological effect. A tragic event can be so overwhelming that, after the event, you may become psychologically stressed or even impaired. This condition is called critical incident stress (CIS).

CIS is any experience that goes beyond what the provider normally deals with. Situations that involve multiple victims, a friend or acquaintance, a co-worker's suicide, severe trauma to the victim's body, a highly publicized event, a rescue that takes an extended amount of

Tough stuff can be dangerous, but it can also present a great opportunity.

time or unusual effort—or even an ordinary emergency call—can result in stress that produces both psychological and physical symptoms.

The CIS concept was pioneered by Dr. Jeffrey Mitchell at the University of Maryland. Dr. Mitchell found that when people have a chance to debrief or talk about a critical incident and their personal feelings under the guidance of a trained debriefing team, the incidences of both short- and long-term stress are significantly reduced. His research has led to a formal practice called critical incident stress debriefing (CISD), in which trained teams conduct a group session for rescuers and EMS workers soon after an event. These teams include trained peer counselors, psychologists, and clergy.

Almost all EMS training programs now include some instruction in stress, including signs, symptoms, and management skills. Debriefing teams have been organized nationwide to assist EMS organizations in conducting debriefings. Specific groups and associations can assist your organization in setting up a team or a debriefing.

Within forty-eight hours of the call in Webster, the responders were invited to come together to talk about the incident. It was a very informal gathering. People talked about what had happened, as well as the loss, their feelings, and their questions. They supported one another and acknowledged that they were dealing with much more than an ordinary call.

With the help of debriefing sessions and the greater awareness such sessions bring, most EMS workers appear to cope fairly well with incident-related stress. "We were debriefing long before we knew what to call it," one long-time paramedic said. "We've always gotten together and talked about the bad calls, but now we do it with less alcohol and more professional help. None of us is saying, 'It's part of the job; it doesn't bother me.' We know better now."

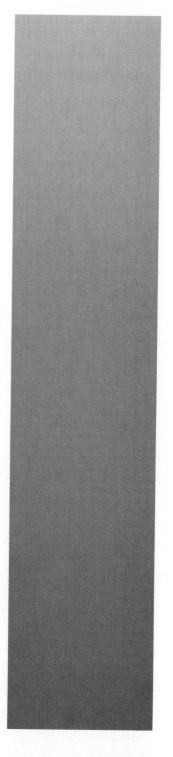

The Other Danger

There is a less obvious danger related to critical incident stress—one that can have a powerful impact on your success in EMS. Dealing with human suffering and death on a daily basis may affect your perspective on life. Your optimism may fade or disappear behind a cloud of cynicism, bitterness, and pessimism.

An example of this is the character of Hawkeye Pierce on the old TV series *M*A*S*H*, set during the Korean War. Hawkeye, a young, life-loving doctor, finds himself in the middle of a confusing war. His daily work is mending an endless parade of battlefield casualties. On the surface, Hawkeye is OK. He doesn't become crazed with stress, fall apart, or quit. He may complain and act zany, but like so many EMS people, Hawkeye has the admirable ability to clean up from one tragedy and move neatly on to the next.

Underneath Hawkeye's quick smile and practical jokes, we see the hint of a hard edge. As the war progresses, his youthful innocence fades away, and his outlook on life begins to take on a pessimistic note. Everything he sees suggests that the world is in desperate shape. In one episode, after a long day of caring for wounded soldiers, Hawkeye tells his fellow doctor, B.J., that nothing seems to matter anymore. Each day is just a blur of senseless tragedies. All Hawkeye wants is to go back home and forget the war. The problem is, he can't forget. His experiences with tough stuff have left a deep, dark impression that will not go away.

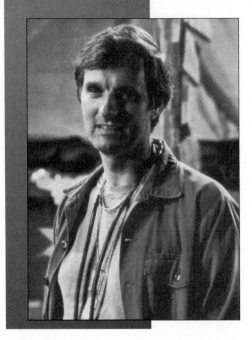

Alan Alda plays Hawkeye Pierce on TV's M*A*S*H. *Underneath Hawkeye's laugh and practical jokes is the hint of a hard edge.*

This is a real danger of tough stuff. After dealing with tragedies call after call, you begin to wonder about life. One paramedic said, "I guess I've just got a screwed-up view of the world now. I used to believe in God. I thought somebody was in charge, but I just don't know anymore. I went on this call where a 14-year-old boy had hung himself in his parents' clothes closet. We were doing CPR on this kid, and his mom comes in and starts bitching about the clothes that had been trampled when rescue cut him down. That call was enough to stop me from believing in a lot of things."

Another paramedic who had worked in a busy EMS system for seventeen years said, "I still do calls because medic work is better than sitting in an office, but I don't have any dreams anymore. I used to think about going to med school or maybe starting my own business. I've seen too much on the street to be a dreamer. Street work makes you pretty practical about life. I guess you could say I've learned that you just take what you can get. There are no good guys or bad guys. We're all just here to see how far we can go, and if you're lucky, you won't get hit by a car."

Another paramedic denied that the tough stuff affects him. "That's all b.s.," he said. "It's just a job. People get sick and hurt, and sometimes they die. So what? The only real stress out here is the idiot drivers. You can't get dramatic about this—it's horizontal taxi work." Yet his statements clearly showed that he had been affected.

The EMS novel *Street Dancer*, by Keith Neely, has a sad, desperate mood about it. The characters become great practitioners. They learn to handle every kind of emergency with great skill, but their personal lives fall apart. Instead of finding satisfaction and joy in their work, they develop a flat, fatalistic view of life.

This is what often happens in EMS work. Taking care of other people's tragedies begins to wear you out. One

> *"The experience of burnout has a particular kind of poignancy. Having started out to help others, we're somehow getting wounded ourselves. What we had in mind was expressing compassion. Instead, what we seem to be adding to the universe is more suffering—our own—while we're supposedly helping."*
>
> —Ram Dass

> *"A great sadness had descended upon him and he could not move or talk or feel."*
>
> —From *Street Dancer*

"We die with the dying:

See, they depart, and we go with them."

—T. S. Eliot

EMS veteran described it this way: "One morning you wake up and find you just don't care anymore. Your skills may be OK, because that's your job, but you don't give anymore. You stop doing the extra stuff. When I first started, I wanted to be the best I could be. I lived for EMS, but now there's nothing special about the work. It's actually pretty depressing. It's like all the stuff you see takes away your life piece by piece."

Little formal research has been done on the cumulative effects of working with other people's tragedies, perhaps because the effects are difficult to assess. The tough stuff gets mixed up with the grind of shift work and the struggles of life outside the job. You begin to feel like your life is going nowhere, that you have no purpose, and that everything is boring, but it's difficult to say exactly what's causing the distress. By looking closely at some of the ways tough stuff affects you, you can begin to understand how this other danger might be managed.

First of all, tough stuff makes you confront death and mortality. You may have signed up for EMS hoping to save lives, but as you go on calls, you rapidly discover that death often wins. Of course, you know death is a natural part of the life cycle. Experiencing life's sudden ending over and over can magnify death so that it seems like life's only destination.

You are confronted with your own mortality. You realize that the person crumpled in the car before you could have been you. As long as you work in

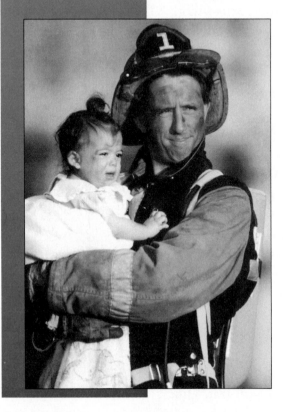

Glamorous photos and posters hide the tough stuff that makes up much of EMS work.
PHOTO COURTESY OF TONY STONE IMAGES, INC.

EMS, you will face a continual and extremely vivid reminder that you are but dust, and to dust you will return.

Second, much of the tragedy and suffering you see defies explanation. The tough stuff will continually raise questions that have no answers. I once went on a call in which a man had been critically injured in a car wreck just moments after his wedding ceremony. The wedding party, in long formal dresses and tuxedos, followed the ambulance to the ED, where the bride, in her bloody white gown, screamed and protested as her new husband was pronounced dead. She climbed onto the ED cart beside him and cried bitterly. "Why, God?" she said. "Why is this happening to me?" But there was no answer, no explanation.

Remember that old black-and-white fire prevention poster of a firefighter carrying a child from a burning building and giving him mouth-to-mouth resuscitation? That poster made sense. But when it was me blowing into the charcoal-tasting mouth of a lifeless 7-year-old boy—the victim of an arsonist's fire—suddenly there was no sense to it.

Tough stuff can make it seem as if the world is out of control, as if the calls themselves are illustrations that there is no plan, that nothing really makes sense, that all is chaos.

The third way tough stuff affects your outlook on life is that it matures you before your time. Everyone in life must eventually face tough stuff. Regardless of what field you are in, you will eventually encounter tragic experiences and face your own mortality. The EMS experience compresses a lifetime of learning into a very short amount of time. You may see more tough stuff in a weekend than most people see in a lifetime. Such experiences are life-changing, and the change is not always good. You can become bitter. Like the boy who goes off to war and comes back a man, EMS will force you to grow up quickly.

This is the other danger of tough stuff—a danger that

> *"To ask "Why do the righteous suffer?" or "Why do bad things happen to good people?" is not to limit our concern to the martyrdom of saints and sages, but to try to understand why ordinary people—ourselves and people around us—should have to bear extraordinary burdens of grief and pain."*
> —Harold Kushner

"It seems like it happened all at once—like I woke up one day and realized my life was a mess. I was getting a divorce, I was alone—a long way from the life I had expected to be living."

—A medic

We always have a choice in how we respond to life.

you will slowly lose the joy and optimism in your work and life. You will become cynical toward your work, your patients, and the world around you. Everything will seem flat and colorless. What once promised to be an exciting and full life will have turned into an empty, hollow joke. Like the tin man who slowly rusts, you will squeak and creak through life wondering why you have no heart.

But this is only a danger. You need not become a victim of the tough stuff in EMS. As we discovered in Chapter One, our lives are not determined by the things that happen to us and around us. We always have a choice in how we respond to life. We can let the tough stuff squash us, or we can choose to see the opportunities in it. We can acknowledge that the tough stuff is indeed difficult. We can allow ourselves to grieve and practice the art of balancing.

Opportunities in Tough Stuff

One of our strongest needs as humans is to find meaning in life. When social scientists from Johns Hopkins University asked nearly 8,000 college students what they wanted most from life, seventy-eight percent said they wanted to find meaning and purpose. The famous psychologist Carl Jung once said, "About a third of my cases are suffering from no clinically definable neurosis, but from the senselessness and emptiness of their lives."

We want to know that life is more than just a short biological event. When we are old and gray, we want to be able to look back over the events of our lives with a sense that living is more than just an exercise in survival. This desire for meaning is what makes us human.

Nothing seems to question life's meaning more than the tough stuff. Responding to a call in which a young woman has been beaten and raped will leave you wondering whether anything in this world makes sense. This type of questioning in the wake of a tragic event is a normal reaction. When we experience tragic events, we question life's meaning. Ironically, it is often in questioning the tough stuff that we discover meaning. Often, something difficult or even tragic must happen before we see what's important. Like the fire used to refine gold or the surgical cut needed to fix a wound, the tough stuff is needed to help us discover what really counts.

The reason that meaning can be found in the tough stuff is because the difficult, mysterious, and tragic things in life lie very close to those things that are beautiful, joyful, and satisfying. The poet Kahlil Gibran described this connection of joy and sorrow when he wrote:

> Some of you say, "Joy is greater than sorrow,"
> and others say, "Nay, sorrow is the greater."
> But I say unto you, they are inseparable.
> Together they come,
> and when one sits alone with you at your board,
> remember the other is asleep upon your bed.

In being reminded of your own mortality and confronting life's difficult questions, you are also presented with an opportunity to discover the value of your life and what really matters. Tough stuff and meaning walk hand-in-hand.

Consider another character from *M*A*S*H*. Col. Potter, the commanding officer of the M*A*S*H unit and a doctor, sees as much tough stuff as Hawkeye Pierce. In fact, being older than Hawkeye, Col. Potter has witnessed the

"What is to give light must endure burning."
—Viktor Frankl

"Crisis is opportunity riding on dangerous winds."
—A Chinese saying

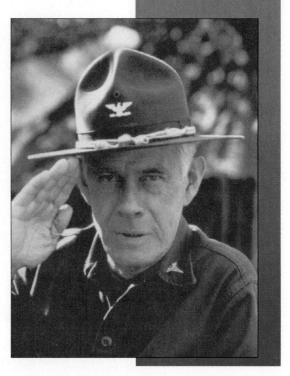

Harry Morgan plays Col. Potter in M*A*S*H*. Even though Col. Potter is in the midst of his third war, he still sees beauty in the world.*

horrors of both World War I and World War II. Yet, his outlook on life is not bitter, cynical, or pessimistic. Rather, he is optimistic and hopeful. He has a calm view of the future.

How is it that Col. Potter finds meaning in the same battlefield experience that overwhelms Hawkeye? The difference is in how they choose to approach the tough stuff. Those of us in EMS have a similar choice to make.

Acknowledging Tough Stuff

In *Platoon*, a dark movie about the meaninglessness of the Vietnam War, there is a powerful scene in which a group of soldiers has returned from a patrol where several comrades died. They are overwhelmed with grief, but in an effort to dull the pain, they stand in a circle with arms around each other and begin to chant, "It don't mean nothin'. It don't mean nothin'. It don't mean nothin'."

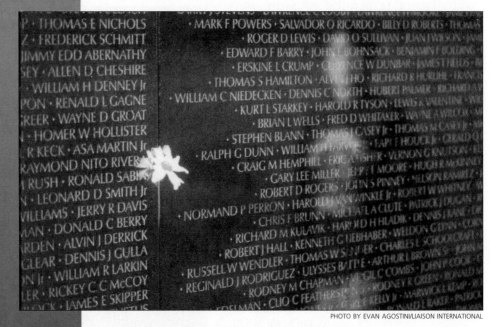

The Vietnam War Memorial in Washington, D.C., is helping the nation heal from the horror of that war by acknowledging those who gave their lives.

It is a moving scene that graphically depicts an attempt to hide from the pointlessness of that war.

But tough stuff—even the tough stuff of a questionable war—can begin to have meaning if it is acknowledged. In the Constitutional Gardens in Washington, D.C., there is a black granite memorial to the men and women who died in the Vietnam War. Invisible from the road, its two wings, stretching 247 feet, are filled with the names of the more than 58,000 Americans who died in that war. As you walk down the cobblestone path, it is as if you are walking into the darkness of the war itself. The emotional impact of that place is powerful. People often weep as their fingers trace the names of the dead.

This memorial is significant because it acknowledges that no matter how awful the war was and how much the nation would like to forget it, it did happen. As that event is acknowledged, people begin to find meaning and to experience healing—meaning in the courage and sacrifice of those who died, lessons in the horrors of misguided government policy, and hope in the prayer that such events will never be repeated.

Many EMS workers fail to acknowledge tough stuff. Because it can be painful to remember and because so few calls are recognized as significant by the media, medical community, or management, there is a tendency to simply ignore the tough stuff and move on. Yet, to deny that you have experienced something serious is to lie to yourself. EMS is full of difficult and tragic experiences. The first step toward finding meaning in the tough stuff is to acknowledge it. You must allow yourself to admit that you are dealing with tragic events.

"Those who do not know how to weep with their whole heart don't know how to laugh either."

—Golda Meir

Try This:

Make your own hall of fame for tough stuff. Think about your experiences in EMS and make a list of the tough calls you remember. Use just a few words to describe the calls, such as

- *C-arrest in the church*
- *Suicide by the lake*
- *Winter accident on Highway 15*
- *Two kids in apartment fire*

As you make your list, notice your feelings. What is it about these calls that makes them memorable? Don't try to find meaning in anything just yet. Simply acknowledge the calls and your feelings.

As you acknowledge the tough stuff from your past and on a daily basis, you may experience troubling questions. Why am I sad? Why did God allow this to happen? What does this all mean? Allow the questions to come. You need not have answers. In fact, you will rarely find concrete answers for such things. The questions themselves will open your mind to finding new meaning.

Acknowledging the tough stuff will often produce strong emotions. Let the emotions come. They are a sign that you are allowing yourself to grieve and heal.

Allowing Yourself to Grieve

You may wonder why you feel sad on certain calls. It seems silly. You don't know the people, and their sicknesses, injuries, or deaths don't really affect your life. You'll go back to the station, then home, and your life will not be changed by their loss. So why do you feel sad? Why do you feel as if you've lost something? You feel sad because every person's loss is also your loss.

There was an old European custom in which the church bell was rung when someone in the community died. People all around the countryside would hear the bell ring and then begin asking, "Who are they ringing the bell for? I wonder who died."

In answer to those questions, the poet John Donne

wrote, "Never send to know for whom the bell tolls; it tolls for thee." Every time we experience a death, we are reminded of our own mortality. When we encounter someone else's tragedy, we feel sad because we can never completely separate ourselves from the plight of humankind.

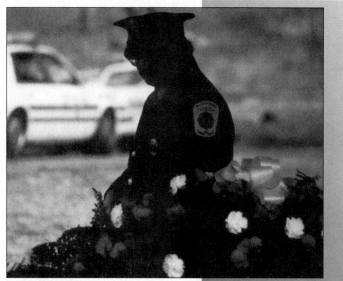

PHOTO BY TOM CARTER

The strong emotional feeling you experience in tough stuff is called grief. Grief is the emotion experienced in the loss of something or someone of value. The feelings you experience may include the entire spectrum of human emotion—anger, fear, sadness, and even hysteria. You allow yourself to grieve when you give expression to these feelings.

Unfortunately, grieving is difficult for many EMS workers. They can sympathize with their patients and comfort family members and fellow workers, but they are often unable to express their own grief. Part of the reason comes from EMS workers' tendencies to care for everyone else. EMS people are accustomed to taking care of others and paying close attention to everyone else's feelings. They often fail to recognize their own.

Not allowing yourself to grieve is like denying a part of yourself. Sam Keen, a wonderful writer on men's issues, says, "When we repress our grief, we blunt our capacity to experience joy." One of the great opportunities of tough stuff is its ability to help you get in touch with your own feelings and perhaps experience a higher degree of joy.

Allowing yourself to give expression to your feelings is a slow process, but it can be learned. At a recent work-

Grief is the emotion experienced in the loss of something or someone of value.

> To feel the pain of another's tragedy is
>
> - Normal
> - Necessary
> - Proof that you are emotionally alive
> - A good sign that you care
>
> Allow yourself to grieve. Don't hide from it or run from it. Just feel it and be with it.

shop on grief, one paramedic said, "I haven't cried in years, and I don't think I want to. So how can I express the way I feel about something I find sad?" The best way to express grief is in whatever way is most natural for you. It's OK not to cry. Pay attention to your feelings. Notice when something bothers you. Take time to feel the emotion. Try talking about your feelings. Find a partner or friend you trust and tell that person how you feel. Give all the details about the event and what specifically bothered you.

Try This:

Return to your list of tough calls from the last exercise. Go over the calls again, and ask yourself if you allowed yourself to grieve. If not, spend some time giving expression to your grief. Don't try to grieve about everything at once, however. Grief is a process that will take its natural course once you allow it to begin.

As you allow yourself to grieve, your emotions will begin to loosen and unclog. As you express your grief about a specific call or situation, feelings and memories from your past may emerge.

Recently, a paramedic told a story about trying to resuscitate a 43-year-old man who had arrested while working in his yard. Obviously, the call was bothering the medic deeply, and he began to express his grief by yelling and swearing about his inability to intubate the man. He continued talking, and his grief took a personal turn. His father had died several years earlier in a similar situation. He had had many disagreements with his father and had not been able to make peace with him before he died. After nearly an hour of talking and a few silent tears, the paramedic finally declared, "I feel like I just vomited my guts out." In a way, he had—he had vomited up long-held grief for his father. All grief, old and new, has to be expressed.

Ignoring your grief blocks your ability to find joy and meaning. In the very expression of grief, you begin to give meaning and value to the loss.

Creating Balance

There's a good lesson to be learned from diabetic patients. Diabetics must maintain a delicate balance between their injected insulin and their blood sugar. A late night, a missed meal, or stress can easily send these patients into shock. The most healthy diabetics are the ones who learn to balance well.

Tough stuff is a lot like insulin. It can help you discover what is truly meaningful in life, but it can also be overwhelming if it's not kept in balance. Like insulin, it can creep up on you when you least expect it, leaving you flat, pessimistic, and wondering why you're doing this work.

Unfortunately, many EMS people respond to tough stuff by working even more. They sign up for more shifts, take extra assignments, and throw themselves back into the work. Granted, being busy can divert your attention for a while and temporarily dull the discomfort of tough stuff. Eventually, however, it catches up.

Balance is created by acknowledging the tough stuff,

"The tears . . . streamed down and I let them flow freely as they would, making of them a pillow for my heart. On them it rested."

—Augustine, from *Confessions* ix 12

Tough stuff can help you discover what is truly meaningful in life, but it can also be overwhelming if it's not kept in balance.

"During the night we went on a job to an apartment fire. We worked this young boy who had been pulled out of the fire and got him back—sort of. His heart was beating when we got to the ER, but he wasn't breathing. We learned later he didn't make it. In the morning, on the way home from work, I stopped at a bakery and bought jelly- and cream-filled doughnuts—a big white box of them. I woke up the kids and we sat on the porch in the bright sunshine and ate dough-nuts and laughed. It was a great celebration of just being alive."

—A medic

allowing yourself to grieve, and knowing when to take a break. After an experience of tough stuff, you need to get away from work and restore your energy and perspective.

For me, this means spending some time in nature and with animals—away from the pressure of pagers and telephones. Other people I know are revitalized by being around their families or by engaging in intense physical activity. Others look to creative expression, such as music or painting. You'll be surprised how allowing yourself to recharge will help you gain a meaningful perspective on the tough stuff. In the long run, you will gain much more energy and optimism by taking the time to balance. You'll also discover how meaningful your work can be.

Try This:

Reflect on your personal history. What sort of activities, places, and situations are comforting and restorative for you? Make a list of things you might do to find balance.

Finding balance also means cashing in on the opportunities of tough stuff. As you step back to balance, you'll find a new appreciation for your own life. At certain times, you'll feel fortunate just to be alive, and your problems will pale in contrast to those you have witnessed. The tough stuff can also give you a wonderful new appreciation for the people you love. Don't hesitate to celebrate such discoveries of meaning.

Tough stuff will never be easy to face. As you become more in tune with your feelings and allow yourself to acknowledge the tough stuff, to grieve, and to balance, your perspective on work will change. A successful EMS worker is not one who learns to go on calls and feel nothing. Rather, a successful EMS worker feels the pain of others and knows that such pain underscores the value of human life.

Summary

✔ Tough stuff is the experience of human tragedy, suffering, and death in EMS work that can impact your success.

✔ EMS deals with a segment of the human experience that our society often avoids.

✔ Tough stuff can be dangerous to the EMS worker.

✔ Tough stuff can produce stress that requires special debriefing.

✔ Tough stuff can change a person's outlook on life.

✔ With a constant diet of tragic events, EMS workers can become cynical and skeptical about life.

✔ There are opportunities in tough stuff for a richer life when the worker does the following:

1) Acknowledges the tough stuff

2) Allows himself to grieve

3) Finds balance between the tough stuff and the rest of life

Suggested Reading

Compassion in Action, by Ram Dass and Mirabai Bush (Bell Tower, New York, 1992). Making sense out of what to do in a suffering world and understanding how to truly be of service to humanity are two difficult issues for EMS workers. An Eastern approach to the ideas of service and compassion, this book is a wonderful journey into what we really do when we help the suffering.

Elegant Choices, Healing Choices, by Marsha Sinetar (Paulist Press, New York, 1988). We heal when we make right choices. Dr. Sinetar shows how the choices we make every day say much about our healing. Even the most simple decisions have profound effects on our lives.

Emergency Services Stress, by Jeffrey T. Mitchell and Grady P. Bray (Brady, Englewood Cliffs, New Jersey, 1989). This application of Dr. Mitchell's work is a valuable resource for understanding the principles of critical incident stress and the process of defusing and debriefing.

EMS Stress: An Emergency Responder's Handbook for Living Well, by Ray Shelton and Jack Kelly (Jems Communications, Carlsbad, California, 1995). This practical guide is written for emergency responders by emergency responders. It is about learning to deal effectively with the everyday stress of being in this work. As the title suggests, it's about living well— healthy and happy.

International Critical Incident Stress Foundation, 5018 Dorsey Hall Drive, Suite 104, Ellicott City, Maryland 21042, (410) 730-4311, Fax (410) 730-4313, twenty-four-hour emergency hotline (410) 313-2473. You can write or call the International Critical Incident Stress Foundation for information on CISD teams in your area or for information on how to obtain training and guidance in dealing with stress in EMS work.

When Bad Things Happen to Good People, by Harold Kushner (Avon Books, New York, 1981). This is a must-read for every rescuer. No one can do this work without asking the questions this book helps answer. Harold Kushner's treatment of this subject comes from a deeply personal experience and yet has practical application for everyone— especially people in EMS.

10 Going Home– Personal Relationships

Love alone is capable of uniting living beings in such a way as to complete and fulfill them, for it alone takes them and joins them by what is deepest in themselves.

—Teilhard de Chardin

A paramedic relayed a sad story while waiting in an idling ambulance on a night shift. Several years earlier, he had met a beautiful woman with auburn hair and a winning smile. Something clicked between them; it was love at first sight. After a flaming romance, they committed to each other in a picture-perfect wedding. Their marriage was going to be different. They were in it for the long haul. But after two children and a few years of marriage, they were separated and planning a divorce.

The paramedic was at a loss to explain what had happened. He wondered if his EMS work had contributed to the failure of his marriage. Would the relationship have fared better if he had been in the insurance or computer business? Was there something more he could have done?

These questions are important for someone creating

> *"The goal of our life should not be to find joy in marriage, but to bring more love and truth into the world. We marry to assist each other in this task."*
>
> —Leo Tolstoy

success in EMS. As he talked about his loss, it became obvious that it didn't matter how successful he was at work. The joy was gone because his marriage failed.

Having a rewarding personal life can be a powerful asset in creating success in your work. EMS asks for a generous heart and a sturdy soul from its workers. Having positive and supportive personal relationships will add a valuable perspective to your work. They will bring new meaning to helping others in crisis.

It's difficult to say how much EMS work will affect your personal life. Everyone comes to EMS with different upbringings, family backgrounds, and personal issues. Considering the nature of the work and the testimonies from those in the field, you can expect that EMS work will have some influence on your personal relationships. But *how* it affects your relationships is largely up to you. Whether you are married, single, gay, or somewhere in between, considering how to blend your work with your personal relationships will add to your success.

Risk Factors

When teaching CPR to laypeople, talking about the risks of heart disease probably saves more lives than teaching people to push on Annie. This is also true for rela-

---

EMS and Relationships

There are no comprehensive studies documenting relationship problems in EMS, but one doesn't need a statistician to notice the high divorce rate and troubled relationships among EMS workers. Look around. Maybe it's just a reflection of our larger society, but almost everyone seems to be having difficulty in this area. The good relationship seems to be the exception rather than the rule.

tionships. You may benefit more from learning about risks and prevention than about skills for a last-ditch save.

The biggest challenge facing any relationship today is learning to live in a society that is experiencing tremendous change in the way it views relationships, family, home life, and work. There are numerous ways to interpret the statistics on failed relationships, but there is no denying that people are struggling. Divorce and breakups touch nearly everyone.

There are many reasons for these changes. The breakup of the "traditional" family, the growing mobility of society, the mounting economic pressures on families, and the heightened expectations people have of relationships are all contributing factors. Many of our rituals and traditions have become passe. Many people lack models for a good relationship. In today's day and age, relationships are at risk—whether in EMS or any other field.

EMS does add to these pressures. There is almost universal agreement between EMS workers nationwide that EMS creates certain risks for a relationship that might not exist in other occupations. Let's consider some of these EMS-specific risks.

The EMS Working Day

Consider the working day (or night) of the EMS provider. Each day is made up of two important components: waiting and going on calls. Waiting sounds great to people who don't do it. To many EMS people, waiting can be sheer torture. Sure, you may be able to rest, exercise, read, watch television, or even sleep. But if you do it for very long, waiting can be much more fatiguing and frustrating than being busy.

The waiting creates problems at home in several ways. If you spend the majority of your shift waiting, you may feel a lack of accomplishment. You arrive home armed with an abundance of energy, ready to tear into some-

> The biggest challenge facing any relationship today is learning to live in a society that is experiencing tremendous change in the way it views relationships, family, home life, and work.

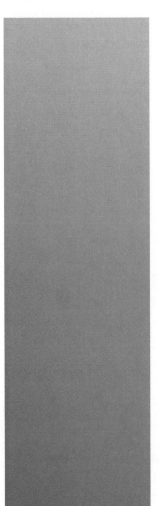

thing useful. After a prolonged period of inactivity, it's difficult to go home and suddenly switch gears.

One medic described going home from a shift this way: "It's like I've got one foot on the accelerator and the other on the brake. I go home and want to get to work—do anything—just so I can feel like I've accomplished something. I'm really energetic at first, but then I tire out and feel lazy. It's like I need a Code 3 call to get me going. I've got a ton of half-finished projects around home and never enough energy to complete them." Such behavior can make a medic very difficult to live with.

To compound the problem, EMS workers often go home with unrealistic expectations and lapse into a frenzied state of getting things done. The spouse of one paramedic said, "If she has a slow shift, she thinks she should come home and do all sorts of work. It's like she feels guilty for not having done much at work. She makes all these promises and lists. Soon she burns out and parks in front of the TV. Then she feels even more guilty. I just wish she'd let herself come home from work and relax like everyone else."

Shift work alone can be a big risk to relationships. Studies show that around-the-clock shift work results in less sleep, a high susceptibility to illness, and a lower level of job satisfaction. All can impact a relationship. Further-

Shift Work

"Shift work is a good place to hide a bad marriage," says University of Nebraska sociologist Lynn White. She has found that shift work, especially night shifts, can negatively affect marital quality. People who work odd shifts are more likely to get divorced than those on regular hours. One of the key reasons White found was shift work brought more jealousy and concerns about faithfulness.

—From *Newsweek*, July 12, 1993, p. 69

more, when couples begin and end their working days at different times, they are bound to have difficulty in coordinating time together when they are both at the same energy level. This can become critical in areas of communication, sex, or just being together.

Night shifts present a unique problem for couples. In many organizations, EMS people are allowed to sleep on night shifts when they are not on calls. After having slept for a few hours at work, the medic will then attempt to begin a day at home as if he has had a full, restful night's sleep. A spouse described the results of such activity this way: "Just because he got to sleep in his uniform at work, he thinks he's had enough sleep for the day. It's like he's afraid to waste the daylight sleeping. I guess he's what you call a type A. He tries to do a bunch of things, but by noon he's so crabby I can't stand to be around him. If I mention getting some sleep, he explodes."

Trying to coordinate a couple or family schedule with an EMS schedule that requires working on holidays and weekends can lead to serious conflict. There is no escaping that EMS work will have an impact on family traditions, holidays, birthdays, and get-togethers. The worker may understand the need to take a turn at working on Christmas, but his family members may not.

The other important element of EMS work is its unpredictability. You never know whether to expect a busy day or a slow one. You may have three slow days in a row and then a shift full of emergencies. It's never just the right amount of calls. Comments such as "it's either feast or famine," "must be a full moon," "had to shoot my partner for

"For the last ten years, we've had to plan our holidays around his schedule. The kids don't really have any Christmas traditions because we can never count on him being home. He's either at work or coming or going. It's a real sore spot around our house."

—A medic's spouse

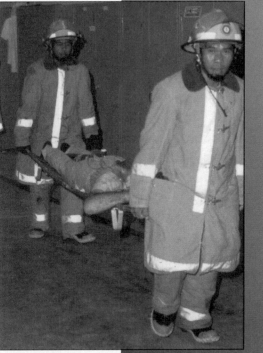

PHOTO BY JOYCE TOMPSETT

a call," or "haven't turned a wheel all night" pervade this work. The people at home can't anticipate your mood.

On your busy days, coming home may be further complicated by the tough stuff discussed in Chapter Nine. When the call load is heavy and the time to absorb is brief, you may bring your frustrations home. Unfortunately, the people who love you may not be able to understand what you've been through during your shift. This "experience gap" can create a barrier between couples.

If your spouse or lover has not done emergency work, there will be things he or she will not understand. Your partner may wonder at your excitement and satisfaction after a "good" call for a bad multiple trauma. He or she may puzzle at the times you come home silent, not wanting to talk about a call, and there will be times when, ethically, you won't be able to say much. He or she will shudder at your dark humor and be baffled by the inside jokes between you and your working partners.

As time goes on, the experience gap grows if the couple doesn't communicate well. You assume that the other person cannot possibly understand your job and the tough experiences you've had. Your spouse or lover assumes that you don't feel comfortable talking, and the silence will grow.

I was once on the other side of an experience gap. I worked with a partner who had been a "grunt" in the Vietnam War and had seen two years of heavy action. Occasionally, he would talk of being shot at by unseen snipers or of walking "point" during a nighttime patrol, but he never really opened up and talked about the experience. There was often a heavy, frustrating silence between us. Because I had not been to Vietnam, I couldn't fully understand. But I needed him to explain more. I needed to know what it was like and how he felt. Our relationship would have benefited from his opening up, but it was his experience, and he had to take the lead in sharing it.

EMS workers often find balance by talking out their

> The people who love you may not be able to understand what you've been through during your shift. This "experience gap" can create a barrier between couples.

frustrations and concerns with partners. If it can't be done during the shift, they will often stick around and talk with the next crew or go out after work with co-workers.

Obviously, this practice can lead to conflict at home. As one spouse said, "Sometimes I really feel left out. If he's had a rough day, he'll go out with his partners after work. It's not like they don't get enough time together. They practically live on top of each other for twelve hours at a time. I mean, it's only natural for me to wonder what's up, why he doesn't want to spend more time with me."

The relationship between partners is often easier than that between spouses or lovers. There is a common shared experience, and partners will often be on the same sleep schedule, an important matter when it comes to energy level and communication. The amount and intensity of time spent with partners often leads to the development of relationships that can be frighteningly close in the eyes of spouses and lovers.

While these are some of the common risks that come with the EMS working day, each organization and situation will present other risks.

Try This:

Every EMS job is unique. Consider the different aspects of your job and the requirements of the position. Make a list of potential risks your job might pose to your relationship. Start with some of the risks mentioned here.

Night shift work: _____

_____

Tough stuff: _____

_____

Extra training: _____

_____

> The relationship between partners is often easier than that between spouses or lovers.

> *"We do not increase our value when we make other people happy, gain people's trust, or provide them with the things they need. [Helpers] do not move up a notch on the 'worth' scale by giving to the poor, protecting the vulnerable, or rescuing those in crisis. The causes for which you fight may be worthy, but they do not increase your worth."*
>
> —Carmen Renee Berry

Money

You've probably heard many times that the biggest conflict in marriage is money. If your primary occupation is EMS, chances are you aren't getting rich. Many EMS workers hold two jobs, and few families are able to get by without both parents working. When budgets are stretched and people are working long hours to make ends meet, there is no escaping the risk to the relationship. The lack of an obvious career ladder in most EMS agencies forces many workers to plan a career change or to squeeze more schooling into an already busy schedule.

Caretaking

One of the greatest risks to personal relationships is establishing the relationship around caretaking. EMS work is centered around the noble virtue of providing care for people in need. Often, EMS workers try to extend their caretaking role to their relationship with their spouse or partner. Such caretaking stifles the relationship, impedes healthy growth, and can eventually be disastrous.

Michael came to EMS work because he enjoyed the fulfillment he received from helping others. He liked being called to crisis situations where he was really needed. After getting into EMS, he fell in love and married a woman named Emily who had two small children from a previous relationship. They seemed to be very happy. Emily, who had been abused in her previous relationship, couldn't believe how kind Michael was to her and the children. He was always willing to help around the house, and he even encouraged her to stop looking for a full-time job so she could stay home with the children. By picking up a few extra shifts and teaching CPR and first aid classes, Michael was sure he could support them all.

Things went fine for a few years. Friends always commented on what a great couple they were and marveled at Michael's willingness to help care for children who weren't his. They complimented his strong dedication to creating a family.

The family grew, and so did the expenses. Michael began working two EMS jobs and still continued to be very involved with the children. He took them to skating lessons and coached T-ball. When the children started school, he asked Emily to look for work, but she didn't want to work. She was out of touch with the working world and enjoyed her home craftwork. Besides, Michael had always been able to come through. He didn't push the issue.

Slowly, Michael began to change. Being a super husband, a terrific dad, and a great medic were no longer satisfying. He needed something else. He began spending more and more stolen moments talking with one of the emergency department nurses. Soon there was more than talking, and Emily finally confronted him. He confessed to being unfaithful, and in Emily's mind the relationship was over.

Michael moved out of the house, but he was confused. He had always thought the real rewards in life came from denying yourself and helping others. Hadn't he taken good care of his family? Why had he been compelled to seek affection elsewhere? What had gone wrong?

Michael had tried to base a relationship on his need to be needed and to take care of others. Instead of creating a healthy relationship, he created dependencies. He had ignored his own need to have a mutual relationship of give and take. Eventually, it exploded.

The tendency of people to extend their caretaking beyond the job can be seen over and over in EMS and other helping professions. In his book *Paramedic*, New York City paramedic Paul Shapiro tells about transporting a young woman with cancer, striking up a relationship, and eventually living with the woman. He cares for her through the terminal stages of her illness until she dies. This may

> The tendency to extend caretaking beyond the job can be seen over and over in EMS.

be a great story of love and dedication, but it also illustrates how EMS people are often unable to separate their need to caretake from their personal lives.

Helping someone is a wonderful act of kindness. But when you begin taking care of a spouse or a lover, you may foster an unhealthy dependency that can eventually lead to problems. There are many psychological explanations for caretaking behavior and its causes, but regardless of the reasons behind it, you must be aware of the tendency to caretake and monitor it in your own relationships.

Try This:

Do you caretake in your personal relationships? Write down your answers to the following questions.

1. *What is your relationship based on?*

    _____

    _____

2. *Are you being "heroic" in your personal relationship?*

    _____

    _____

3. *Do you find it easy to express your needs and have them met?*

    _____

    _____

4. *Do you try to establish a position of power in the relationship by doing things for the other person?*

    _____

    _____

5. *Do you often feel taken care of by your lover or spouse?*

    _____

    _____

6. Do you consider your relationship equal?

_____

_____

If you suspect you are creating or involved in a caretaking relationship, now is the time for some outside input and personal counseling.

Managing Risks

CPR training has been extremely successful in helping people survive heart disease, not only because they learn to manually circulate blood in sudden cardiac arrest, but also because they become powerfully aware of the risks that might lead to heart disease. Being aware of the risks is the first step toward managing a problem. Conquering any obstacle starts with acknowledging that the obstacle is there.

Plan some quiet time with your spouse or lover and go over your list of risks together. Discuss the effects EMS work might have on your relationship. You'll be surprised at how misunderstood your work is by someone because of the experience gap. Describe how you feel when you come home from work. Don't be afraid to talk about the frustrating part of waiting and night shifts. Don't neglect to talk about the tough stuff. Teach your spouse or lover about your job and how it can affect your moods and responses. Together, you can create management strategies.

When a conflict or problem comes up in your relationship, being aware of the risks will help you recognize that there may be something beyond the immediate issue. The husband of one paramedic was concerned that his wife occasionally called at the end of a shift to tell him that she was going out with co-workers. He was suspicious and hurt that she did not prefer to be with him. As they discussed risks, he became more sympathetic to her need for some informal release after a difficult shift.

Teach your spouse or lover about your job and how it can affect your moods and responses. Together, you can create management strategies.

"In a true healing relationship, both heal and both are healed."

—Rachel Naomi Remen, M.D.

Bruce, a paramedic, and Carol, a bank employee, experienced repeated disagreements and conflicts when Bruce would come home after a long shift. Aware of the pattern, they decided to schedule a several-hour "buffer period" after Bruce's return. During this period, Bruce was free to feel and do whatever he wanted. He agreed not to commit himself to chores until after he had time to unwind and get some sleep. They agreed not to discuss major issues during this period. Nor would they put pressure on each other to be intimate.

Carol also agreed to value Bruce's work even if he had spent a shift without any calls. Bruce began to expend his after-work energy by exercising instead of slamming things around the house. The buffer period became a planned part of Bruce's working schedule. Both felt a new respect for themselves and for their relationship.

In some EMS organizations around the country, couples have begun to get together with other EMS couples. Their purpose is to help spouses and lovers learn more about how EMS providers deal with their work. Spouses get a glimpse of the frustrations, fears, wacky humor, and love co-workers share with each other. They also get a chance to compare notes with other spouses and lovers and gain insight into their common experiences.

Try This:

Plan a get-together with several EMS couples. Make it an informal gathering in a comfortable setting. Invite people with the understanding that you want to talk casually about EMS and relationships.

You can begin the conversation by asking if people think EMS work has an effect on relationships. Use the points in this book to stimulate discussion. You'll be surprised at what surfaces.

Addressing risks and real problems helps us stop blaming ourselves and others for the difficulties we experience. Out of risk recognition and awareness, understanding emerges. In understanding, we gain the ability to forgive ourselves and others for not being perfect. As you begin to understand the way you are and why your relationship might stumble over small things, you can begin to see beyond the daily stress factors and learn to enjoy the comfort and pleasure of your relationship.

Signs and Symptoms

When a heart is starving for oxygen, it signals its need with some very specific signs. Hurting relationships also signal their trouble. People who have serious relationship trouble often describe common symptoms that precede a breakup. These symptons signal the need for action. Some signs and symptoms are

1. Silence. "Something was wrong. The thing we enjoyed most when we first dated was talking. We still talk about who will go to the store and when the house payment is due. Except for the necessary stuff, we don't talk anymore, at least not to each other."

2. Apathy toward making the relationship work. "I've stopped trying to make it work. I don't even know if I want help for the relationship. When I think about talking about it, I don't have the energy."

3. Frequent nonspecific anger toward the other. "Inside I feel this raging anger. I don't even know what I'm mad about, but it seems like everything she does makes me furious. I can't even talk without blowing up."

4. Seeking affection outside the relationship. "Little by little, I found myself needing and seeking attention from someone else."

5. A growing feeling of hopelessness about the relationship. "I made a big mistake with this marriage. I know I would have been much happier with someone else

> Out of risk recognition and awareness, understanding emerges. In understanding, we gain the ability to forgive ourselves and others for not being perfect.

or just being alone. I don't see how anything can change to make me believe that we can make it."

The persistence of any of these danger signs is a signal for some serious action. Just as with heart disease, denial is common when it comes to relationships. Even though you recognize the signs, you may deny that they could be anything serious. Often people will say, "Yeah, we've got some problems, but it's not that bad. We'll work it out with time." Or, you may become paralyzed with guilt. People thought you had the perfect relationship, that you were just right for each other. Now you don't want to admit failure.

Relationship problems rarely go away without intervention. If you recognize any of these signals, you need to take action. At a minimum, set aside all other distractions and give serious attention to your relationship. Try to honestly identify the problems without blaming the other person. Then try to develop a plan for resolving the issues. It is imperative that you both agree on what the issues are and how to resolve them. If you can't agree, you will need outside help.

The decision to seek counseling is often looked down on. "What's a counselor going to do for us?" you might say. "I don't want to start going back over my childhood. I don't think a counselor will help." These concerns reflect a healthy suspicion about someone else solving your problems. The truth is a counselor cannot fix your relationship. Rather, a counselor can help you identify what's really wrong and how you might fix it. You will need to do the work yourself. By beginning counseling, you are making a commitment to work on the relationship with guidance from an outside expert.

Don't make the mistake of assuming you can't afford counseling. Relationship breakups and the aftermath will cost you much more than the cost of counseling—ask anyone who's been through it.

Relationship problems rarely go away without intervention.

To find a good counselor, begin asking people you trust to recommend someone. Your minister, physician, and even crisis phone lines can help you with referrals. Find a counselor who comes with strong recommendations and is professionally qualified. This means the person should have training in family therapy, as well as the appropriate certifications and licenses. If possible, find someone who is experienced in working with EMS people.

Once you've identified a counselor, you'll need to assess whether he will work for you. Talk with the counselor on the phone first, briefly explaining why you are looking for help. If the counselor doesn't have time to talk on the phone, then he is too busy to help you. Keep in mind that EMS workers usually need a counselor who has some flexibility in scheduling and who understands the demands of the work.

When you go to your first session, don't expect instant help. Good counseling takes time and effort. Continue to assess the counselor by considering the following:

- Do you feel safe with this person?
- Are you and your partner both comfortable with this person?
- Do you feel like this person listens?
- Do you feel understood?
- Do the counselor's style and general view of life fit yours?
- Does this person believe he can help you?
- Is this person willing to let you make choices?
- Do you both agree that this person might help?

First counseling sessions usually consist of getting to know each other and discussing the nature of the problem. After that, the counselor will begin to help you identify specific problems and plans for dealing with them.

One distraught paramedic had gone to a counselor with her lover and afterward said, "Well, that was a waste of money. I expected her to give us a lot of stuff to work on, but she didn't tell us to do anything." Often, counseling will not provide you with an immediate plan of action, so give it time. Keep your questions in mind and surrender to the process.

In recognizing the signs and symptoms of trouble, you may conclude that there's no hope for your relationship. You may even want it to be over. It's not uncommon for people in caretaking relationships to sabotage the relationships so they can escape from them. Even if the relationship does end, don't neglect to talk with a counselor. The breakup of a relationship is a big loss that will lead to a grieving process. Your self-doubt may be lessened by counseling, even if it only confirms what you already know.

Ingredients for Success

Books such as this can provide you with a great deal of information. Often, they are like new products for spine immobilization—great at addressing the need but way too cumbersome and complicated for practical use. In creating success in your personal relationships, you need something that is easy to use and gets the job done.

In the Midst of a Breakup

- Allow yourself to grieve.
- Your sorrow is a symbol of love's value.
- Be gentle with yourself.
- Find support—this burden needs other helping hands.

There are three essential ingredients in a successful relationship.

Commitment to the Relationship

Several years ago, one of my sons was upset at his inability to hit a baseball as well as others on his Little League baseball team. While he wasn't really that interested in baseball, he was interested in hearing the cheers of his teammates instead of the silence that followed his strike-outs. We discussed how he might improve his batting through practice and set up a schedule to practice every night.

The first night went well; he had great fun hitting the balls while I chased them. The next night his efforts weren't quite as enthusiastic. The third night he declined to practice, as he did again on the fourth night. We sat down for another talk.

"What about the cheers of your teammates?" I asked.

He was silent.

"You can become a good hitter if you just practice," I encouraged.

He looked down at the ground, thinking about the work involved. "I guess I really don't want to hit that good," he said. He had been committed to the rewards but not to the extra work.

A couple happily nearing their fiftieth wedding anniversary, told of numerous difficult times when finances, hard work, and childlessness threatened to tear their relationship apart. During those rough periods, they had to retrace

"Take time to love . . . it is the one sacrament of life."

—From *The Treasure Chest*

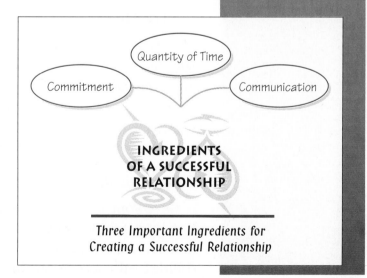

INGREDIENTS OF A SUCCESSFUL RELATIONSHIP

Three Important Ingredients for Creating a Successful Relationship

their path and reconfirm their commitment to each other. This reconfirmation, they said, was the only thread that held them together.

In discussing relationships, people often mention changes, passages, and transitions, but perhaps the most important questions in a relationship are the following: How committed am I to making this work? Am I just in this for the good times? Am I willing to work at this?

"Commitment is the foundation, the bedrock of any genuinely loving relationship," says Dr. M. Scott Peck in *The Road Less Traveled*. He points out that commitment is critical to solving problems in relationships. "Couples cannot resolve in any healthy way the universal issues of marriage—dependency and independence, dominance and submission, freedom and fidelity, for example—without the security of knowing that the act of struggling over these issues will not itself destroy the relationship."

One marriage counselor noted that his clients always profess to being committed to the relationship but often call it quits when the going becomes difficult and their commitment requires personal growth.

Try This:

Assess your commitment to your relationship. To what extent are you committed? What personal changes are you willing to make for the sake of the relationship? What are you unwilling to change for the relationship? How do you express your commitment in your relationship?

Communication

Everyone in EMS knows the value of communication. Not long ago, I responded to call on which everything that could go wrong went wrong. A semi-trailer truck had collided with several cars and then rolled over on top of one. Soon after arriving on the scene, my partner and I became separated. When I reached for my portable radio, it was gone. My patient was in serious trouble, and I needed a suction unit. As I tried to yell for help, the gasoline engine of a Hurst tool roared to life, and I was left trying to manage an airway with my hands. In those desperate moments, I found myself thinking about the importance of communication and all the awful things that can go wrong when it breaks down.

Communication in a relationship is easy to overlook because we are often fooled into believing that talking about daily activities will be enough. To be fulfilling, relationships must consist of more than just surviving together. After being with someone for a while, we often think we know everything there is to know about that person. This is never the case, especially if both parties are growing. There is always more to be learned.

In his book *Love Must Be Tough*, nationally known family psychologist Dr. James Dobson says he thought he communicated well with his wife until his communication skills were challenged at a retreat for married couples. He quickly realized that he had not tapped the depth of his relationship. He described this new learning about his wife as being one of the most meaningful and growing times of their relationship. He learned things about her that had completely escaped him in years of marriage.

For EMS people, an important part of communicating is learning to listen with an open mind. Gathering information during a secondary survey requires listening, but this is listening for specific things that will trip switches, such as heart disease, seizure medications, or recent injuries. Listening to a lover is very different. It requires letting go of the trip switches and opening the mind.

Just relax and listen without looking for the hidden clue. Your relationship should not be a mystery. Communication is an art that is developed and improved with

An important part of communicating is learning to listen with an open mind.

practice. It requires an ear as well as a mouth, and ultimately has great benefits for the heart.

Try This:

Set aside a special time with your spouse or lover to communicate beyond the review of daily activities. A useful technique is to pick a topic and then separate for a period of time to write your responses. Then come back together and read your responses to each other. Let your conversation go from there. Try to make the session respectful and supportive of each other. Here are some sample topics:

The part of me you know least is . . .
When I think of a good relationship, I think of . . .
When I'm old and gray, I want to look back at my life and say . . .

Quantity of Time

We live in a world where many people are preoccupied with saving time. In traveling, cooking, or assessing trauma patients, we are always looking for ways to do it faster. We have to be careful not to make the mistake of applying time-saving techniques to the wrong things. It still takes three months to grow a big watermelon, nine months to make a healthy baby, and years to build a rich and fulfilling relationship.

Each year I seem to get busier and busier, but I've discovered that a good relationship still takes a quantity of time if it is to remain satisfying. A good relationship can survive busy schedules for a while, but it eventually demands the return of a proportionate amount of time. While much has been said about quality versus quantity time, the two cannot be separated. Time together cannot be left to chance. Rarely will you be committed or have

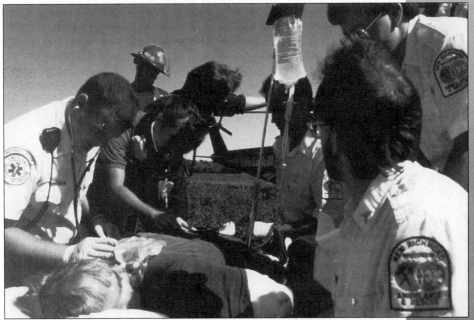

PHOTO COURTESY OF LIFE LINK III

clear communication if you do not invest time in your relationship.

Commitment, communication, and time together build a platform of respect, which is the basis of a satisfying relationship. You may admire, feel sorry for, be turned on by, or be a caretaker of someone else, but you will not be satisfied if there is no respect. Respect grows from making a commitment to someone and appreciating that person as a unique individual.

Anyone who participates in street resuscitation has thought about the difference between a beating heart and a successful life. Just getting the heart going doesn't guarantee that the patient will walk out of the hospital to have a successful life. Similarly, in relationships there is a big difference between survival and success. Many people today choose mere survival and yet, deep inside, hunger for more. One of life's greatest pleasures comes in sharing your life with another.

Commitment, communication, and time together build a platform of respect, which is the basis of a satisfying relationship.

EMS may pose some unique problems to your relationship that require attention and care. It is this attention to your relationship that will help you discover why you work so hard to preserve this thing called life.

Summary

✔ EMS does have an effect on your personal life.

✔ Shift work, night work, and the nature of waiting for calls all affect the EMS worker's responses at home.

✔ The economics of working in EMS can have an effect on personal relationships.

✔ The caretaking nature of EMS work is not a good model for personal relationships.

✔ The risks to relationships can be managed.

✔ There are specific signs and symptoms of relationship trouble.

✔ The ingredients for successful relationships include the following:

1) A commitment to the relationship

2) Good communication

3) Quantity of time

Suggested Reading

Getting the Love You Want: A Guide for Couples, by Harville Hendrix, Ph.D. (Harper Perennial, New York, 1988). Here is one of the best books available for understanding your relationship and making it something special. The book has some theory but is also filled with exercises proven to strengthen relationships. The material has been presented across the country and has been beneficial to many couples.

Ten Laws of Lasting Love, by Paul Pearsall (Simon and

Schuster, New York, 1993). Most of us don't just want an average relationship; we want one that is exceptional. In this book, Dr. Pearsall presents ten principles for transforming a routine relationship into the sort of intimate partnership that endures.

When Helping You Is Hurting Me, by Carmen Renee Berry (Harper Paperbacks, New York, 1988). This book helps people—pleasers, rescuers, givers, counselors, and crusaders—learn to love themselves and put their helping of others in proper perspective. This book is another essential read for EMS people. The desire to rescue is not always noble, and the author puts it into a realistic, healthy perspective.

Who's on Top, Who's on Bottom: How Couples Can Learn to Share Power, by Robert Schwebel (Newmarket Press, New York, 1994). This provocative title belies the trouble that many couples have in creating lasting intimate partnerships. Using case studies, the author presents the reader with some highly practical methods for resolving the power struggle that so many couples have.

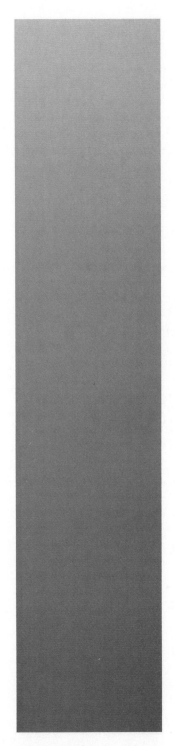

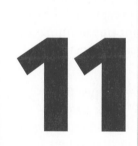

The Art of Comfort

In the midst of all my pain and fear, I suddenly realized I was not alone.

—An EMS patient

Recently, while reflecting on my success in EMS, I looked at a stack of thank-you notes and letters I've received from patients over the years. The file is small considering the thousands of calls I've made, but the small number makes them all the more precious. I noticed that very few of the cards mention my expert medical care, my unwavering skill at starting IVs, or even my ability to read a monitor. Instead, these grateful patients mentioned things such as kindness, helpfulness, and reassurance. They used words like "comfortable," "confidence," and "patience" to describe how my partners and I had treated them.

Perhaps it's not really so surprising that patients and their family members notice the nonmedical care we give. While we are trained to stabilize broken bones, medicate asthma attacks, and shock quivering hearts, the bulk of EMS street work is comforting people in crisis situations and helping them with acceptance, decision making, and entry into the medical system. The most universal need you will find among your patients is not for oxygen or morphine or even transportation. The most universal need is for comfort.

Undoubtedly, one of the most brutal awakenings of street work is discovering the severe limitations of medical science. Medicine cannot change social ills, reverse the aging process, or prevent death.

This realization can strike in a dramatic way. A new medic recently told me of one of her first calls. It was for a boy who had been hit by a car and had an open skull fracture and obvious brain injury. In minutes, the boy was boarded and on his way to the hospital. The medic knew there was little more she could do in the face of such a horrendous injury, but the realization was difficult for her. "I had come to expect I could save anybody who wasn't cold and stiff," she said. "What a surprise it was to sit there bagging that kid while his pupils dilated and his pulse slowed. I felt cheated."

Your medical bag of tricks is limited in what it can fix or change. Yet, no matter what the problem, your patients and their families can benefit from being comforted. There is more to emergency care than the medical protocols. When you comfort, you step beyond the traditional scope of medicine and treat your patients' emotional and spiritual needs. Unfortunately, however, traditional EMS training includes little on the art of comforting people.

What Is Comfort?

Comfort is the easing of pain or unpleasantness. It is like a large, soft pillow when we are weary or tired. A pillow cannot induce sleep, nor can it fix problems or take away worries, yet somehow it makes things just a little bit better. It will cushion and support the head and aid in relaxation. Comfort is a pillow for the soul. It may not change circumstances, give hope, or alter the outcome, but it can cushion the pain and unpleasantness.

"When and where did we lose sight of the fact that the last word in EMS is 'service'?"

—James O. Page

There is more to emergency care than the medical protocols. When you comfort, you step beyond the traditional scope of medicine and treat your patients' emotional and spiritual needs.

Comfort/
kŭm´ fərt/ n.
state of physical
or mental well-
being or
contentment;
relief of suffer-
ing or grief,
consolation;
person or things
that give this.

—*Oxford Dictionary
of Current English*

Emergency—
any condition
that the person
requesting
assistance
perceives to be
an emergency.

—*Federal EMS
Program definition,
1973*

Comfort is conveyed through human interaction. It is having an empathetic human being nearby and knowing that the person cares. People often choose their personal doctors based not on their medical credentials or diagnostic skills, but on how they treat their patients and make them feel. People are concerned about whether their doctors are comforting—whether they are kind, understanding, unhurried, and willing to talk with their patients. And while your patients cannot choose who will help them in an emergency situation, they need the same characteristics and responses from you.

Try This:

Stop and consider your own feelings about comfort. Consider a time in your life when you experienced pain, sorrow, a crisis, or a loss. Think about your interactions with other people during that time. What was comforting? What seemed to cushion the unpleasantness?

In the current climate of efficient, cost-effective, assembly-line EMS, such characteristics are typically not emphasized, primarily because they cannot be measured easily in a quality program. This doesn't negate their importance. In fact, many large EMS operations could benefit from rethinking their concepts of customer service. Instead of focusing on response times, loaded units, and technical medical gadgetry, they may do better to look at customer service in terms of *comfort*.

The problem is, learning to comfort is not as easy as reducing response times. Comforting another person is a human act that emerges from who you are, coupled with your attitude about people and yourself. Everyone has his own style and method of comforting, but there are three important ways you can become a comfort to those you are called to help. They are

- Being a compassionate presence
- Acknowledging the situation's importance to the patient
- Being an active resource

Being a Compassionate Presence

One of the most enduring childhood memories I have is of my mother sitting up with me at night when I was sick. For a number of years, I had strep infections at least three or four times a year, which in turn brought me every flu bug that existed. The nights were always difficult; my fever would spike, and I'd become nauseated and would vomit. Patiently and kindly, my mother would stay up with me until I drifted off to sleep. And when I awoke, as if by magic, she would hear me and return to my side.

Interestingly, my mother had no special powers to reduce my fever, take away the pain, or stop the nausea, yet her mere presence made me feel better. To this day, whenever I'm sick, it's her presence I miss and long for most.

The hardest part of any crisis is feeling frightened and alone. When we experience a loss, a difficult situation, an injury, or an illness, we feel cut off from others. Our patients experience the same feelings of fear and loneliness in the midst of their crises. Something unpleasant and unknown is happening to them. Beyond their physical discomfort, they feel a sense of confusion about what is happening and why they've been singled out for this calamity. You can help ease their discomfort by being comforting, which simply means being a compassionate, reliable, and gentle presence. This can be done by communicating in a calm, confident voice and offering a reassuring touch.

Imagine going on a call for a middle-aged man who is having an MI for the first time in his life. The man is in pain, he's short of breath, and he's extremely anxious.

> *"We shall never know all the good that a simple smile can do."*
>
> —Mother Teresa of Calcutta

> *"I would rather make mistakes in kindness and compassion than work miracles in unkindness and hardness."*
>
> —Mother Teresa of Calcutta

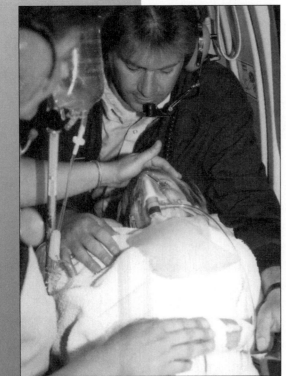

PHOTO COURTESY OF LIFE LINK III

Certainly you want to perform a thorough medical assessment and tend to the needs of oxygenation, pain relief, and ectopy treatment. But you can comfort him at the same time. Start your assessment by introducing yourself. Then shake the patient's hand or touch him on the shoulder. Such an introduction not only conveys that you are an expert there to help, but that you are also a fellow human being with a name. As you begin to assess the problem and gather information, inform the patient that you'll be staying right beside him. Keep your voice calm, and explain your actions.

On the way to the hospital, take a moment and convey your presence by doing something more than the medical procedures. Talk with your patient, wipe the sweat off his forehead, make sure the pillow and blankets are adequate, and touch him in a reassuring manner. Don't hesitate to address his fears.

I often ask people if they are afraid, and they typically nod yes or even acknowledge some specific fear. I don't try to answer or counter their fears, but I do agree that chest pain, car accidents, and uncertain futures are indeed frightening. Just listening to someone's fear can be comforting to them. When the fear is voiced or named, it somehow loses some of its power. You don't need to give false hope or some profound explanation for your patient's crisis; just listen and then assure him again that you'll be staying beside him and doing the best you can.

There is no right or wrong way to do this. You will develop your own style, and as long as you attempt gently and compassionately to convey your human presence, you'll be successful.

Acknowledging the Situation's Importance to the Patient

In three successive 1991 issues of *JEMS*, publisher Jim Page tells about two EMTs who transported his elderly aunt to the hospital. Her condition necessitated ambulance transportation but was not life-threatening. According to the medical need, the EMTs may have performed acceptably, but their attitude toward their patient was one of complete indifference. It was just another call for them. They ignored her, talked over her, and completely failed to acknowledge that this call was significant to her.

Almost anyone who has spent time on the street can understand the actions of these EMTs. Working the streets, you deal with crisis every day. It becomes easy to see each call as just another run, especially if the patient is not critical. Yet, each call is important to the person you've been called to help, and treating a patient's crisis as unimportant and bothersome can make your patient feel worse than he already does. On the other hand, acknowledging the situation's importance by paying attention to the patient and talking with him can be very comforting and reassuring.

Recently, I responded to an elegant supper club where a very distinguished-looking man had become nauseated and passed out in front of a large group of friends and acquaintances he was hosting for dinner. The man was awake and feeling better when we arrived and apparently had just had a little too much to drink before dinner. My partner and I could have treated the man and his crisis as if it were nothing and just left. After all, he didn't want transportation, and we had both seen countless drunks from all walks of life and were not impressed by the setting or his fancy suit. Yet, in an effort to provide more

Each call is important to the person you've been called to help.

"Sure my EMS forms are hurried and messy. What really matters is if I've talked to my patient. Any system that tries to take me from spending more time with the people who need my help is not focusing on what counts."

—A medic

than just a medical service, we assisted him from the club and let him sit in our ambulance while awaiting a taxi. We recognized the situation for what it was for the man— a tremendous social embarrassment.

Several days later, our organization received a warm letter from the man expressing how comforting it was to have such help during his crisis. We had performed no medical wonders, but we had succeeded in comforting the man by acknowledging that the call was indeed important to him.

The same principle is true for situations in which you have medical concerns about your patient. People take great comfort in knowing you are taking their situation seriously. It's important to express your concern about your patient's condition. Let him know that you recognize that this is important. Contrary to the media-magnified problem of ambulance abuse, most patients feel embarrassed about calling an ambulance and admitting their need for help. Validating their crisis is comforting to them.

Being an Active Information Resource

Several years ago, I went rock climbing with a group of eager and experienced climbers. I knew nothing except my desire to scale an enormous rock face was matched by my fear that I might fall onto the rocks below. The experienced climbers talked among themselves about "belaying" each other, about "free climbing," "bouldering," and "carabiners." They squinted up at rock faces, arguing about whether they were "5-8s" or "5-9s." It was all a foreign language to me and did little to boost my faith that the nylon rope tied to a harness around my waist would keep me from falling.

Many of your patients and their families will feel much the same when confronting medical technology. While they may have watched Johnny and Roy and seen a few real emergencies on tabloid television, they will largely

Questions a Patient Has in the Midst of a Crisis

- What's happening to me?
- Who are you and what are you doing?
- Can you help me?
- Where are you taking me—what's it like?
- Am I going to be all right?
- Am I dying?

"This year, about twenty-five million Americans will be transported in ambulances. Yet only about ten percent of them will require emergency care to stabilize their conditions or restore vital functions. If our EMS culture glorifies those cases while virtually ignoring the remaining ninety percent, can we be satisfied?"

—James O. Page

be uninformed about what's happening and what you're doing to them, not to mention the outcome. To you, this will be just another call—a minor trauma, angina, a faker, or a low back—and you will automatically swing into your routines and protocols. Your medical lingo and procedures may be disconcerting to the patient. In pausing to explain, you can provide a great deal of comfort.

As you begin to care for your patient, explain what you're doing and why. Emergencies are wonderful "teaching moments." The patient is very concerned about how he is feeling and what you can do about it. Your explanations can be simple, yet comforting. Tell why you're putting on an oxygen mask: "This will help give your heart the oxygen it needs and may ease the pain." Explain the need for the IV (many people think IVs are for nourishment when they can't eat): "This will provide us the best way to give you medicine." Help them understand why they need to go to the hospital: "We want to make sure you're OK, and we can't perform enough tests here to determine exactly what's wrong."

On the way to the hospital, briefly describe the destination and what will happen once your patient gets to the emergency department. Of course, you can only speak in generalities, but any information is extremely helpful. I usually say something like, "We'll be at the hospital in several minutes, Mrs. Anderson. The medical center is a big place, but the emergency department really does a good job. When we get there, the nurses will repeat many of the same things we've done here. They will ask you several questions, and one of the doctors will examine you. They'll probably take some X-rays and blood tests. Do you have any questions?"

In presenting yourself as an information resource, you are providing a level of comfort patients desperately need.

In many EMS services today, the emphasis is on turn-around time and getting out of the ED and back on the street as fast as possible. This has led many medics to use their transport time to write their reports. Except for glancing at vital functions and the monitor, they virtually ignore their patient. Such efficiency may speed your return to the street, but you will have missed an important part of caring for your patient. Those few moments you spend in the back of the rig can be either anxiety-producing or comforting for your patient. If you take the time to be a resource, you will not only help your patients, but you will also have the successful feeling of truly having made a difference.

Comforting at the Death Scene

The call was for a man down. My partner and I had a bad feeling about the run and found a 52-year-old man on the kitchen floor. The first responders were doing CPR. As I entered the room, I noticed a woman looking on from the next room with wet eyes. With a quick look, my partner found a nonperfusing slow rhythm. I quickly secured an ET tube and an IV and pushed in an amp of epi. CPR continued, but the rhythm soon stretched out into asystole. We tried more epi, but nothing changed. I quietly conferred with the medical control doctor and decided it was best to quit. As I hung up the phone, I glanced to where the woman had been standing, but she was gone.

> If you take the time to be a resource, you will not only help your patients, but you will also have the successful feeling of truly having made a difference.

She had disappeared into the living room, probably suspecting what I was about to tell her.

What do you do at a scene like this? How can you continue to help people when your medical skills have failed to save the patient? The death scene is perhaps one of the most difficult calls you will face in this work. You've been trained to save lives, but what about that inevitable job of telling someone a loved one is dead? And what about you? Of all your calls, the death scenes will be some of the most intense.

For a number of years, I had the privilege of leading a grief support group. I heard grieving people talk about death scenes and the importance of those few moments surrounding the death. While many medics underestimate their role in these situations, they are extremely important and can leave a lasting impression on the patient's loved ones. By gaining a deeper understanding of grief and your role in the death scene, you can provide a valuable service for grieving people while enhancing your own perception of success in a situation in which we often feel only failure.

Understanding Grief

Grief is the emotion or combination of emotions we experience whenever we lose someone or something dear to us. Grief is the actual feeling of loss, but it is also a journey or process that can last for months and perhaps even years. It is the process by which we acclimate to the loss, reframe our view of life, and move on; it is the process of working through the loss both intellectually and emotionally. There are three sequential stages to the grief process: the crisis or the ending, a "wilderness" period, and a period of new beginnings.

The crisis or ending stage begins when the actual loss occurs or at the moment the news of the loss is announced. The period lasts from several hours to several

> *"To grieve is to embark on a journey not of our own making. It is a journey that is both perilous and unpredictable."*
>
> —Leonard and Hilary Zunin

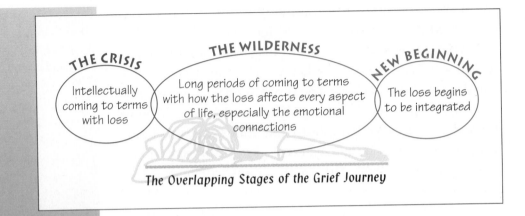

THE CRISIS

Intellectually coming to terms with loss

THE WILDERNESS

Long periods of coming to terms with how the loss affects every aspect of life, especially the emotional connections

NEW BEGINNING

The loss begins to be integrated

The Overlapping Stages of the Grief Journey

weeks, until the grieving person comes to an intellectual acceptance of the loss. For many people, the loss is a seemingly unbearable nightmare, a bombshell going off in their world, especially if the loss is unexpected. During this stage, the grieving person must keep reminding himself of what has happened, as waves of emotion wash over him again and again.

Talking about the death of her sister, one woman described her crisis this way: "After crying all day, I finally fell asleep. Then suddenly I woke up. I knew something was wrong, but it took me a few minutes to remember. And then I remembered in a rush—Clara's dead. I was overwhelmed with emotion, like I'd heard it for the first time all over again."

The crisis also includes a period of deliberate activity in which the grieving person plans and participates in important ending rituals, such as the wake and funeral. During this period, people often seem to pull themselves together because their activities are planned and structured around specific rituals. Frequently, the mourners will be composed and appear to be doing quite well at the funeral. They will appear to be coping, but often this composure is simply a response to all of the activity surrounding the loss.

Once the funeral is over, the relatives return home, and the grieving person settles back into everyday life, something unexpected happens. He wants to get on with life, but a curtain of darkness has dropped. He has accepted the loss intellectually and wants to get on with life but can't. The aching in his heart will not go away, and the world seems empty and full of pain. The person feels as if he will never be happy again, as if the sun will never shine as brightly as it did before the loss. This is the wilderness stage of grief, a confusing time filled with profound sadness and emptiness.

Imagine a telephone operator sitting at an old-fashioned switchboard, with dozens of wires plugged into her control board as she switches calls from place to place. Suddenly, a bully comes along and in one sweeping motion jerks the wires out of the board. It's a shock, but it doesn't take the operator long to realize she's been disconnected. The blank board and dangling wires are sufficient evidence. But getting back into service presents a problem. She'd like to plug the wires in as fast as they were pulled out, but reconnecting is a slow, tedious process. She must pick up one wire at a time, find its place, and then plug it in, pick up another, find its spot, and plug it in. Slowly, one at a time, she reconnects herself.

This is what happens in the wilderness of grief. The grieving person wants to recover from the loss, but there's no way to reconnect all of the emotional strings that have been broken. It is a slow process of reconnecting the strings one by one. The process can take months and sometimes even years. Some people never get over their loss and wind up being permanently lost in the wilderness.

The journey out of the wilderness is slow. As people begin to reconnect with life little by little, they begin to notice new beginnings. Unexpectedly, they catch themselves enjoying something. Gradually, the ache in the heart seems less severe. Of course, they'll go back and forth

> *"In the moments after a crisis, we are stunned as we seek to comprehend what has happened. The very first words that are spoken are usually "I can't believe it."*
>
> —Robert Veninga

"In the midst of winter, I finally learned that there was in me an invincible summer."

—Albert Camus

between the wilderness and new beginnings, but slowly they gain ground. Completing the journey of grief is not to forget the loss. Rather, it is to become reconnected and realize that the loss is not the end of life, but a change, albeit a very painful, permanent one.

As a medic, you will have an important impact on your patients' journeys of grief because you will be present at the sad beginning. You can ease the pain a little by lending comfort.

Comforting in the Crisis of Grief

Remember when the Space Shuttle *Challenger* exploded? That awful moment is etched in our memories. I remember exactly where I was when I heard the news: I was at home, just sitting down to read the paper, when my oldest son burst through the front door. He was out of breath and could only utter the words, "It blew up. It blew up." At first I thought something had happened at the neighbor's house, but finally he was able to convey enough that I turned on the television. Over the next hour, we silently watched the replay of those dividing smoke plumes arching across the blue sky. Most of us will never forget that scene.

People seldom forget the

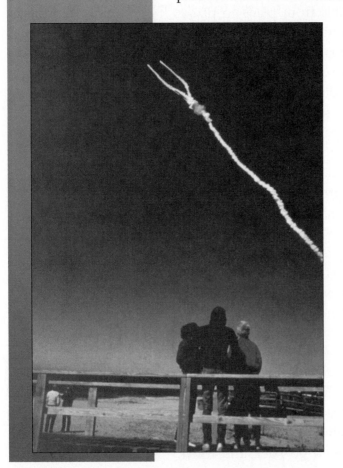

The awful moment of the explosion of the Space Shuttle Challenger is etched in our nation's memory.

moments surrounding a major loss. In the grief support group mentioned earlier, people often talked extensively about the events surrounding the deaths of their loved ones, and I was amazed at how well they remembered everything, even the very words people said. Those moments become a mental videotape grieving people play over and over. They remember what happened, the things said and done, and how they felt. It's as if everything surrounding the loss is magnified in their memories. Frequently, they talk about the actions and attitudes of medical people, including EMS providers.

Since what happens at a death scene and how it is coordinated will be remembered vividly, EMT workers should do everything possible to make sure the scene is respectful and focused on the needs of the grieving friends and family. You can be comforting by taking a leadership role and coordinating the events surrounding the death. Begin by showing care and concern for the body of the deceased. Of course, out-of-hospital deaths will be coroner cases, but, in most situations, this will not stop you from covering the body with a clean sheet and clearing the room of excess rescue people and gawkers. Speaking to one another in quiet, hushed voices will be appreciated. It may be your third death scene of the day, but remember, this is an overwhelming event for those who are grieving.

Your role will also be that of a medical authority speaking for the medical community. This role is extremely important to the grieving, for in our culture, death is largely seen as a medical event. Thus, the loved ones need to hear the announcement of death directly from you. Remember that their need in the crisis is to come to an intellectual acceptance. They need an honest, direct statement of what has happened. They may already know or suspect the truth, but they need to officially hear the words from you. Be gentle, but direct. I usually say, "Mr. Smith,

> Do everything possible to make sure the scene is respectful and focused on the needs of the grieving friends and family.

we've done all we can. I'm sorry, but she's gone." You may need to repeat it and say it in a different way. "Her heart has stopped, and there's nothing we can do. She's dead." I usually try to touch them on the shoulder when I make this announcement. Sometimes my voice is shaky and emotional, but the important thing is that they hear the official medical word.

When you are attempting a resuscitation and know you'll be discontinuing the effort, prepare the family first. With CPR still in progress, take a moment and tell them things are not going well, that you can't get the heart started, that it doesn't look good, and that you'll be trying for a few more minutes. Once you stop the resuscitation efforts, immediately tell the family the news. They of course suspect what you're going to say, but they still need to hear the words.

Try This:

Imagine you are at a death scene and it's up to you to tell the family their loved one is dead. What will you say? What specific words will you use? Words such as "he's gone," "she's passed away," and "he's dead" are all acceptable and direct enough, but find words that work for you. Don't skirt the issue by trying to find a poetic way of telling the family without having to say the words directly. Convey your empathy by your tone of voice, your touch, and your general attitude toward the scene. There is no way to soft-pedal death.

Practice what you will say by saying it out loud. You may discover you are uncomfortable saying these words even in practice, but it's better to prepare now.

Initial reactions to the news of a death can vary greatly, and there is no right or wrong response. There may be silence, crying, anger, hysteria, confusion, guilt, or com-

> "There is no grief like the grief that does not speak."
> —H. W. Longfellow
>
> "Give sorrow words; the grief that does not speak
> Whispers the o'er-fraught heart and bids it break."
> —Shakespeare
>
> "Concealed grief has no remedy."
> —Turkish proverb

plete disbelief. All responses are acceptable as long as people don't try to hurt themselves. Great wailing, crying, and screaming are acceptable and, in fact, are good signs. Such outbursts show intellectual acceptance and a healthy expression of feelings. Rescuers and bystanders often feel uncomfortable with such expressions and want to sedate the grieving person, but don't. There is no need to sedate someone unless the person is in clear danger of harming himself, in which case he should be taken to a crisis center for an evaluation.

If you see people trying to hold their emotions in, encourage them to let them out, and don't be afraid to hold them while they sob. The crisis stage of grief is one place where hugs are still acceptable. Some people accept the news stoically, with very little reaction at all. This, too, is acceptable; just make sure they understand what you've told them.

After you've delivered the news and the loved ones have reacted for a few moments, get them to talk about what just happened—even if they're crying. Gently (without acting like you're investigating) ask what happened. When did they last see their loved one? What did she do today? How did they find her? Had she been sick? Your purpose here is not to investigate, but to get the victim's

"All I need is for you to sit with me. When I cry, don't try to stop me. When I curse God for allowing this to happen, don't defend Him. When I ask you to tell me the details again, please do it. Don't try to cheer me up. Don't tell me about God's reasons. Don't tell me heaven needs him more than I. Just sit with me— I may cry all night long."

—A grieving mother

loved ones to interact with the event that has just happened. They will come to a better intellectual acceptance of what has happened by talking about it. There is no way you can force them to think about anything else, so you might as well talk about what's on everyone's mind: this terrible thing called death.

Often the bereaved will stop in the middle of an explanation and say, "I just can't believe this. I can't believe this is happening. We were going over to the kids' house today . . ." and their voices will trail off as they once again realize how much this loss will change their world. Gently ask another question and help them find their way back to what they were talking about.

Confusion is a common characteristic of people in a crisis. During a crisis, people find that their concentration crumbles and thoughts jumble, and they have a difficult time focusing. Their conversations wander. Don't offer any spiritual or philosophical explanations to people in this situation. If they ask, "Why did God let this happen?" you need not have an answer. Simply agree that this is very difficult and is hard to understand.

People often respond to tragic news with a powerful feeling of guilt. They may blame themselves for not calling sooner, for not having encouraged their loved ones to live healthier lives, or for not being better people themselves. This is almost always the case with parents in the sudden death of a child. You can be of great comfort in these cases by countering their expressions of guilt by saying, "These things happen, and you can't blame yourself. There was nothing you could have done that would have changed the outcome." For some reason, such obvious declarations have a powerful influence when said in the midst of a crisis.

Ask the family if they would like to see their loved one. If it's not a crime scene—and if possible—prepare the body by placing a pillow behind the head, closing the eyes and mouth, and covering the torso and extremities. Even if the deceased has been traumatically killed or horribly dismembered, let the family see if they want to. This is contrary to popularly accepted practices, but the grieving person's imagination of the injury will in time become much worse than the reality. They will only take in as much as they can, and seeing will certainly not deepen their grief.

Prepare them for what they'll see and then accompany them to the body. Often, seeing the body will produce a new wave of emotion, but it will also have a positive effect in helping them accept the reality. They may want to kiss the body or grab it, cling to it, and sob. This is all acceptable. It's their death scene and their loved one. Even if you're uncomfortable, you don't have the right to orchestrate the scene for your comfort. It's their comfort that matters.

Recently, I arrived at a call in which a man was in asystole. We stopped resuscitation efforts, and I went into the living room to tell the family. A 16-year-old son couldn't believe his dad was dead and wanted to see for himself. I led the boy to his father's sheet-covered body, with his mother and siblings following close behind. As soon as he saw his dad lying there on the floor, he yanked off the sheet and grabbed his father's shoulders. "Dad, you can't do this to me," he yelled. "We've got work to do. You promised me we'd go hunting this year. Dad, come on now, snap out of it." We let him go, and finally he collapsed on top of his father's bare chest and sobbed. The rest of the family crowded around, and soon everyone, including the rescuers, had wet eyes. The boy's expression gave the rest of the family permission to grieve. They all sat on the floor around the dead man and began to talk about what a great father and husband he had been.

The police officers and rescuers were uncomfortable at first. It was certainly not a textbook death scene, but after watching, no one there doubted that it was the right thing to do.

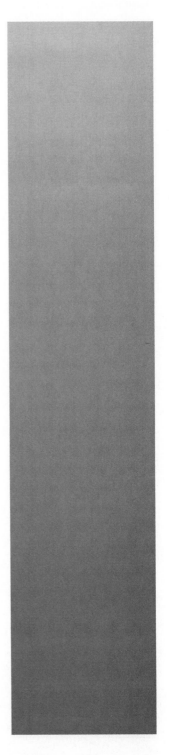

> ### *Resource List for Death Scenes Should Include*
>
> - A chaplain who is comfortable with death scenes
> - Several members of the clergy who are willing to respond to death scenes
> - Crisis centers that can provide crisis counseling over the phone
> - Community service volunteers who can provide transportation and child care
> - Social workers who can provide information on community services
> - EMS physicians who can provide in-depth medical explanations

Every EMS service should have a list of resources you can call.

Finally, you will comfort the family by assisting them with support resources they need during the first hours of the crisis. Because the grieving person or persons will need to make important decisions at a time when they are overwhelmed with disbelief, confusion, and disorientation, support is essential. Even little things, such as choosing a funeral home, can be a monumental decision in the midst of a crisis. You can help by assisting the family in calling other family members or a chaplain. Offer to help and, since you may not be able to remain on scene, make the first order of business finding other support resources. Every EMS service should have a list of resources you can call. An important rule of thumb is not to clear a death scene until reliable support for the family has arrived. In some places the police will take care of finding support, but don't assume.

Before you leave the scene, give the family your name and your EMS organization's phone number and tell them to call if they have any questions. They may not realize until later that they want to ask you what you found when you arrived or whether the loved one said anything before he died. It is a comforting gesture that says you're interested in their loss.

Death scenes can be some of the most rewarding calls in this work because it is there that you will find yourself connected to the circle of life, community, and human compassion. I once responded to a late-night death of an old German farmer's wife. She had been dead for some time before we arrived, so we did a quick check and pronounced her. The old farmer couldn't believe she was dead. Over and over, he said he was supposed to die first; she was younger and healthier than he, and they had always talked about his dying first. His disorientation was profound.

My partner, Gary, could not reach the man's pastor, and the farmer's son was en route, but was several hours away. The sheriff's deputies left for another call, so my partner put us out of service, and we sat down at the kitchen table with the man. He asked if we would read from the Bible, but when I opened the big, black book, I found it was printed in German. For the next hour we just talked. He told us all about his wife, how they met, their life together, and the son they lost in the war. Occasionally he would break down and cry, and every few minutes he would get up and go into the other room to look at his wife's body—just to be sure. Finally, someone from the funeral home arrived, and a few minutes later, his son walked in.

As Gary and I headed back to our station, we both felt immensely grateful for our work, for in our effort to comfort the elderly man, we, too, had found great comfort.

> *"Nobody will ever know about most of the things you do for people—nobody except them and you. Nobody will ever need to know, because that's what makes you a rescuer. It's what makes you special. No, not special—a treasure."*
>
> —Thom Dick

Summary

✔ One of the most important needs of your patients is comfort.

✔ Comfort is the easing of pain or unpleasantness through human interaction.

✔ The three important ways one comforts in EMS are by

  1) Being a compassionate presence

  2) Acknowledging the situation's importance to the patient

  3) Being an active information resource

✔ The moments surrounding a death scene are critical for the grieving family.

✔ Grief is the process or journey of coming to terms with a loss.

✔ There are three stages in the grief journey:

  1) The crisis

  2) The wilderness

  3) New beginnings

✔ The medic's role during the crisis stage of grief is that of coordinator, medical authority, and comforter.

Suggested Reading

The Art of Condolence, by Leonard M. Zunin and Hilary Stanton Zunin (Harper Perennial, New York, 1991). What do you do for people in the aftermath of a tragedy or death? This helpful book will give you a lot of guidance in developing your comforting skills.

The Gift of Hope: How We Survive Our Tragedies, by Robert L. Veninga (Ballantine, New York, 1985). This book describes the grief journey as well as how people can travel the grief journey with a positive outcome. Full of first-hand accounts, it provides a great education in what will comfort.

How to Survive the Loss of Love, by Melba Colgrave, Harold H. Bloomfield, and Peter McWilliams (Bantam Books, New

York, 1976). This small book has helped many through a dark night.

On Death and Dying, by Elisabeth Kubler-Ross (Collier Books, New York, 1969). Anyone who is around death and the dying should read this book. Even though it has been around for twenty-five years, the book is still invaluable for understanding the process of death and how we accept it. This book has material that will be valuable not just for EMS but for all of life's journeys.

Transitions: Making Sense of Life's Changes, by William Bridges, Ph.D. (Addison-Wesley, Reading, Massachusetts, 1980). This book is the standard in the study of how people cope with life's big changes such as the loss of a loved one.

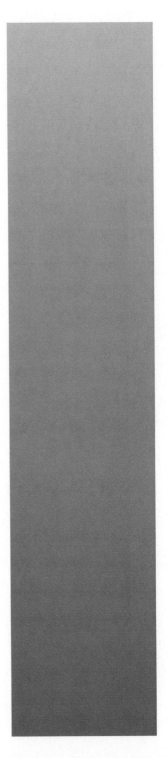

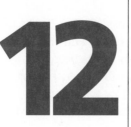

12 | Preparing for the Long Haul

That which we persist in doing becomes easier—not that the nature of the task has changed, but our ability to do it has increased.

—Ralph Waldo Emerson

Congratulations. You're on the road to success. No matter where you might be on your EMS journey—at the beginning, at a crossroads, or climbing a big hill, you're on the way to shaping your own unique success in this work.

Now that you've started, you're probably wondering about the future. What lies ahead? How long can you expect to do this work? Is it possible to remain satisfied and challenged for a long period of time?

When I began in EMS nearly twenty years ago, people told me that EMS is a young person's job. They said, "Do your time and then move over and let someone else have a turn." They talked about the physical demands of the job, the limited pay, the career ceilings, and the tragic nature of the work as important reasons why EMS could not be a long-term career. Indeed, many people do leave the field, but now that modern EMS has been around for a while, we're also finding that many people stay for the long haul.

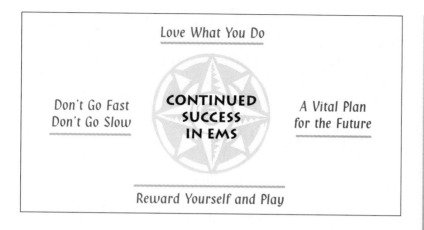

Two questions will inevitably arise as you consider your future in this work:

- How can I remain successful in EMS over the long haul and not become burned out or unhappy with the work?
- When is it time to leave EMS?

How you answer the first question will have a great influence on the second. If you don't create personal success in EMS, you will not want to stay. Furthermore, if you don't create success in the field but stay anyway, you'll find yourself joining the ranks of unhappy and frustrated EMS workers.

This book has attempted to help you answer the first question through ideas and concepts based on actual EMS experience. It's important to remind you that creating success over the long haul will not be easy. In fact, maintaining success in this field requires attention, personal discipline, and diligence. It requires being true to yourself and reminding yourself of your own personal mission.

A growing number of EMS people are creating enduring success in this field. In fact, many people are shaping their EMS work into lifetime careers. Nationwide, more and more people with years of EMS experience are staying in the field without burning out or becoming cyni-

Many people are shaping their EMS work into lifetime careers.

cal. As you look at these successful people, you'll notice that they share some common characteristics and attitudes about their work: They love what they do, limit how much they work, continue to grow, plan their futures, reward themselves, and enjoy themselves.

Loving What You Do

A relationship with EMS work is much like a new romantic relationship. In the beginning, you are powerfully attracted to EMS; you have a gleam in your eye as you respond to your first calls. You look as if you've just fallen in love. You can't get enough. You want to talk about EMS, dream about it, and even wear it on your belt. You probably say, "I just love this work." It's easy to find success and fulfillment because you feel good about the work.

Just as in romantic love, your feelings begin to change. What was once exciting and mysterious because it was so new, becomes more routine. As this change takes place, the flaws become more obvious, the irritants begin to surface, and what was once a magical, thrilling experience becomes commonplace and perhaps boring. It becomes easy to pick apart the work and criticize it for not living up to its early promises. You begin to wonder if it's time to leave.

Most EMS workers—including the successful ones—experience this change in their relationship with their work. Trying to maintain the exciting edge you felt on your first call is like trying to maintain the feeling of a first date throughout the relationship; it just doesn't work. But successful people recognize that this change is not fatal. They also realize that as the relationship changes, they have to work harder at loving the work. One paramedic described it this way: "When I first got out of training and on the street, I was a certified adrenaline junkie. I couldn't wait to see what the next call would be. But after a while, things got pretty routine. Once I'd seen a lot of emergencies, the thrill began to wear off. I started to blame the job, the profession—everything but myself. But that wasn't the end. It's taken a while, but I'm learning that my work can still be a great experience—I just have to invest more in it."

Attitude is extremely important. When you wake up one morning and see EMS with all its flaws and short-comings, you know it's time to put something back into the relationship. You have to love what you do.

To love your work is more than a feeling—it's an active process. You have to choose to love the work in spite of your changing feelings. Ellen, an EMT and paramedic for twenty-two years, described how she loves her work. "It all depends on what you're looking for," she said. "If you're just looking for EMS to please you, you're in for a big surprise. A lot of EMS people expect the work to be like entertainment. When they discover themselves on re-runs, they start complaining and saying what a terrible job they have, and then, of course, it becomes a self-fulfilling proph-ecy—a real drag. I have to put personal energy into my work to get personal satisfaction from it. If I make an investment, really put my heart into the work, regardless of how I feel at the moment, I get something out of it. I don't just wait for the job to make me happy."

Lasting success requires a personal investment in lov-ing what you do. And to love what you do means having pride in your work and believing in its worthiness. It means recognizing the value of your labor and those things that originally attracted you to the work.

Several years ago during a period of doubt about my EMS work, I was cleaning the house and came across an old EMS calendar that was full of dramatic, glossy EMS action pictures. While I enjoyed thumbing through the pictures, I wouldn't have thought of hanging such a cal-endar in my house because I didn't want to glorify my work. Like many other EMS people, I had developed an

> *"Man's main task in life is to give birth to himself, to become what he potentially is."*
> —Erich Fromm

> To love your work is more than a feeling—it's an active process.

How to Love What You Do

- Speak highly of your work.
- In your thoughts, value your labor.
- Perform your duties with great care and reverence.
- Celebrate your daily accomplishments.
- See your work through positive eyes.
- Trust your decision to be in this work.
- Give your best to the work.

attitude of trying to portray my work as just another job (although deep inside I didn't believe it). I threw the calendar away.

My 8-year-old son found the calendar in the garbage. He took it to his room, cut apart the pictures, and taped them up on the wall. Later that evening as he was preparing for bed, he called me into his room to admire his work and ask me questions about the pictures.

"Boy, Dad, is this really what you do at work?" he asked.

"Well, sort of," I replied, not wanting to play up the dramatics. "It's usually not that big of a deal."

He paid no attention to my minimalizing the work. "Have you been to car wrecks like this?" he asked, pointing to a picture of a bad accident scene.

"Sure," I said, remembering such a call just the day before.

"How about this?" he asked, moving to a picture of EMS people hunched over a patient and a cardiac monitor. I'd been there, too.

And on it went. For almost an hour, I looked at my work through the honest, wondering eyes of an 8-year-old. After we had talked about all the pictures and he had asked dozens of questions, my son looked up with eyes full of pride and said, "Boy, Dad, you have a really neat job."

Suddenly, my work did look like a pretty special job. Seeing it through the eyes of a child made me realize that what had become ordinary and routine was something important. I realized I was doing the work I had always wanted to do—work that was meaningful to society and that made the world better. It wasn't just a job.

Seeing real value and worthiness in the work you do is critical to your success. Give yourself permission to say on a regular basis, "This is good work." Actively love what you do. Just because a manager, a patient, a partner, or the community may not value what you do doesn't mean that it isn't valuable. Trust that your choice of an EMS career was correct. You were drawn to this work, so value it and invest yourself in loving what you do.

Try This:

Regardless of the value society places on your work, make a list of the things you value about what you do in EMS. What do you find redeeming about the things you do? What makes this work unique compared to other occupations?

_____

_____

_____

_____

_____

_____

Don't Go Fast, Don't Go Slow

This Zen axiom is a perfect prescription for maintaining success in EMS over the long haul. Successful people

> Seeing real value and worthiness in the work you do is critical to your success.

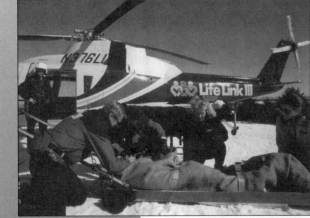

PHOTO COURTESY OF LIFE LINK III

Take a step back and see the value and worthiness of what you do.

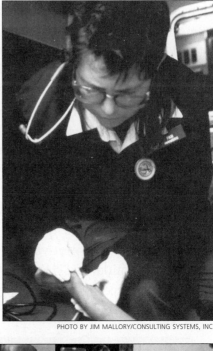

PHOTO BY JIM MALLORY/CONSULTING SYSTEMS, INC.

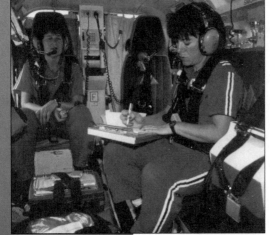

PHOTO BY PETER ESCOBEDO

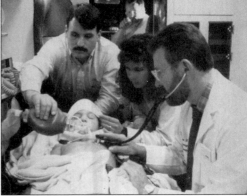

PHOTO COURTESY OF LIFE LINK III

don't go fast, and they don't go slow. They stay in motion but maintain balance and continue to grow.

We live in a society that is chronically out of balance and plagued with addictions. Everywhere you turn, people are addicted, are recovering, or are trading one addiction for another. But one of the most subtle and yet perhaps most destructive addictions is workaholism. In her book

The Overworked American, economist Juliet B. Schor points out that many of us become caught in the "squirrel cage of work and spend." In other words, no matter how much we work and make, it's never enough.

Seventeen EMS people who have been in the field for at least ten years recently were asked how much they are working today compared to ten years ago. None said they are working less; four are working about the same, and the rest are all working more than ever. Furthermore, many are working multiple jobs, and some are even working two full-time EMS jobs. One person is an EMS manager who still feels the need to work a second job.

The need for more money is the reason most EMS people give for working so much. One paramedic explained, "I need to work two jobs. With a couple of kids and a mortgage, I need the income. I know I'm burning myself out," he said, "but I just don't see any way around it."

Such thinking and justification are short-sighted. In her book *Working Ourselves to Death*, management consultant Diane Fassel writes, "Everywhere I go, it seems people are killing themselves with work, business, rushing, caring, and rescuing. Work addiction is a modern epidemic, and it is sweeping our land. . . . I call it the cleanest of all addictions. It is socially promoted because it is seemingly socially productive. . . ."

Work addiction is common among people in EMS. Because of the long shifts and twenty-four-hour nature of the job, it's easy to work more than a full-time schedule and fool yourself into thinking you're getting ahead. Furthermore, in many EMS circles, being exhausted from having worked extra shifts seems to be a badge of dedication. In fact, it's not uncommon to hear EMS people brag about how many shifts they work in a week. Ultimately, the result of overworking will take you far from the success you had hoped to find in selecting an EMS career in the first place.

"The trouble with life in the fast lane is that you get to the other end in an awful hurry."

—John Jensen

Successful people don't go fast, and they don't go slow. They stay in motion but maintain balance and continue to grow.

LOSS OF ENJOYMENT
LOSS OF PURPOSE
LIMITED FINANCIAL GAIN

SPECIAL SIDE BENEFITS:

Chronic Exhaustion, Back Injuries,
Fatigue and No Social Life

The BIG Payoff for Overworking in EMS

During my early years in EMS, I became a workaholic. I worked multiple jobs and taught classes on the side, all in the hopes that I would eventually get ahead financially, and in the process, get recognition for my efforts. Neither happened. No one really noticed all my work, and my reward was chronic exhaustion. As I paid my bills, the extra work became meaningless because in working so much, I lost sight of my purpose, goals, and perspective. Sixty- to eighty-hour weeks were common, and I justified my workload by pointing out that I could occasionally sleep at work if I wasn't on calls. But there was no escaping the sheer number of hours, and as the years ticked by, there was no payoff.

When you work too much, several things happen. First, the work itself ceases to be enjoyable. It's like ice cream or amusement park rides—an overdose destroys the joy. When I limited my EMS work to forty hours and committed myself to not working extra shifts, my enjoyment of the work suddenly improved. I once again looked forward to going to work, and I found myself enjoying the calls and the community with my co-workers. I once again began to take a deeper interest in my patients and wanted to contribute to the EMS field in general.

Second, in working too much, you lose sight of your goals. One of the most tragic things that happens among many EMS people is that they lose the focus of their goals and purpose. When you are chronically exhausted from working too much, interrupting your sleep and trying to squeeze in some play time between jobs, you don't have time to dream or to plan. Tired EMS people are always singing the "I don't know what I want to do" blues, because dreaming and planning for the future take time and energy.

Third, in the long run, you will probably not make financial gains by simply working more hours. An interesting thing happens as you try to deal with financial problems by simply putting in more hours: As the candle burns at both ends, the situation usually becomes more hopeless and you feel the need to reward yourself for all your hard work. So you spend more, and the cycle of work and spending begins to feed its insatiable appetite until you are completely exhausted and still no further ahead.

Why is it that the people who work the most are the ones who also seem to have the most financial problems? Could it be that in working hard, they are not working smart?

People who are successful in EMS over the long haul don't go fast; they limit their work. They recognize that a full-time job is just that—a full-time job! They practice moderation in extra EMS activities, knowing there is a heavy price to pay for overdoing it. It's wise to limit your EMS work to about forty hours per week. In some cases in which twenty-four-hour shifts are worked, people seem to do all right working more, but as a general rule, working more than a full-time job in EMS will greatly diminish your success.

This advice goes against the way many EMS organizations are run. In fact, many EMS operations nationwide expect people to work an unhealthy number of hours and justify it by allowing them to sleep between calls and during night shifts. As professionals who want to be successful in this work, we need to assert ourselves and help organizations correct their use and abuse of EMS workers.

Beyond limiting how much you work, slowing down means relaxing and recharging your emotional, spiritual, and physical batteries. Successful people recognize their need for time and activities in which they are not caring

"Money doesn't talk; it swears."
—Bob Dylan

Slowing down means relaxing and recharging your emotional, spiritual, and physical batteries.

"It is time for us to break free of our overly serious approach to life and laugh, have fun, cultivate frivolity and joy. We (helpers) need to learn how to say "Yes!" to having fun, to going on adventures, to attending spiritual retreats, to spontaneous outings, to developing our artistic talents, to listening to music, to reading enjoyable books, to soaking in bubble baths, to exercising regularly, to filling our homes with cut flowers and beauty and art."

—Carmen Renee Berry

for others. They do not compromise their own need for recreation because of a staffing shortage or a special project. They recognize their need to play and be renewed.

People rarely grow old wishing they had worked more. Rather, they often regret that they did not take more time for things other than work. In his book *When All You've Ever Wanted Isn't Enough*, Rabbi Harold Kushner tells of one 85-year-old woman from Kentucky who said, "If I had my life to live over again, I would dare to make more mistakes next time. I would relax. I would be sillier, I would take few things seriously . . . I would eat more ice cream and less beans."

We need to eat more ice cream in EMS. We need to relax more and have more fun. Our EMS work should be a lot less like *Hill Street Blues* and more like *M*A*S*H*. Look at the people who are creating successful lives on a daily basis. Are they strung out, always grabbing at their personal pager, rushing to pick up an extra shift? Or are they the ones who take the time to laugh, enjoy themselves, and celebrate what they do?

Don't go fast!

Try This:

How do you relax and recharge your batteries? Make a list of things you enjoy doing that don't involve work or taking care of others.

_____

_____

_____

_____

_____

_____

Now look over your list. How many of these things have you done this week?

Do you schedule relaxation and time off with the same determination that you schedule work? Make a schedule for the next month in which you give the same priority to time off the job as you do to time on the job.

The other part of the Zen prescription for success is, "Don't go slow." In EMS, it's easy to get into the field, learn your skills, and then sit back and react. Yet nature teaches that whatever is not growing is dying. Muscles that are not used will eventually atrophy. Even though EMS is noisy, full of action, and sometimes very intense, it also can be passive work in which people stop growing and challenging themselves. Craig, an experienced paramedic, described it this way: "Once I got through the first couple of years, I found myself just sitting around and waiting for calls. I did well on my calls, but other than that, I spent most of my time sleeping or watching TV. I think I've seen every episode of *Cheers* at least a half-dozen times. For a while, I knew the characters on *Hill Street Blues* better than my partners. One day, I realized I was doing the same thing at home; it was just like work. If something urgent needing doing I did it, but otherwise, I didn't have any energy. I was dying. I was tired all the time. I didn't have any ambition at all."

It's easy to get lulled into a comfortable pattern in which you cease to develop. But successful people control this tendency and continue to grow. They look for ways to challenge and improve themselves and their relationship to their work.

Craig describes the difference challenging and improving himself made in his outlook: "The police department was looking for medics to go through training with their SWAT team, so out of boredom, I signed up. It was a really challenging course both physically and mentally. I learned a lot, but more important, I found a new interest in my paramedic job. In the end, SWAT work wasn't for me, but through that, I realized I needed to grow. I started taking a few classes at the university and am now working toward a degree. I've become involved in the CQI [continuous quality improvement] program at work and now have an opportunity to say how things are run. My workdays don't drag anymore, and I enjoy my job more than ever."

Staying in motion and growing are as important as not overworking. In his course "Enriching Your Job," motivator and industrial psychologist Frederick Hansen says, "Personal growth and development are essential to finding satisfaction in work. Even in the difficult times, if a person is growing and developing, he will enjoy a higher degree of fulfillment and satisfaction."

There are many ways you can continue to grow both in and outside of your EMS work. There are the traditional opportunities of becoming involved in supervision, management, or education. There are also more personal ways of developing through taking classes or simply disciplining yourself to develop a new proficiency.

Some of the happiest people in EMS are those who practice vocation/avocation. This means that they use EMS as a vocation, or a means to earn their living, while also practicing an avocation, such as art, music, computers, writing, or raising horses. This combination seems to benefit both their EMS work and their avocation while the contrast between the two enhances both.

How you grow depends on you, but the secret is in recognizing the *need* to grow. Think about the last time you learned something new or expressed yourself in some unique way. How did that experience make you feel? When you grow, you awaken a powerful, creative force within yourself. You start seeing opportunities instead of barriers and you begin to move forward on the road to success. One of the most powerful ways to begin growing is to create a vital plan for your future.

A Vital Plan for the Future

Thinking about and planning for the future may not be a comfortable experience. But there's a big difference between planning and worrying. The third characteristic of people who create ongoing success in EMS is that they plan for the future.

Making a Plan for Your Current Work

Your current work refers to what you are doing right now as well as what you will be doing in the next five years. In relation to your work, where do you want to be professionally in five years? What do you envision yourself doing? By looking five years ahead, you begin to give yourself enough time to prepare and accomplish the sort of things you want to do. If your desire is to be a manager, educator, or administrator, it may take this long to prepare. If you're considering using your EMS experience to go on to nursing, medical school, physician's assistant school, the fire service, police work, or an entirely different field, five years is certainly not an unusually long planning and preparation time.

A plan helps you begin to see how the things you're doing now can affect tomorrow's success. Instead of feeling like you are stagnating, you could be building something you really want.

Planning in EMS work is more important now than ever as EMS faces some of the biggest changes it has seen in two decades. In

> *"Long-range planning does not deal with future decisions but with the future of present decisions."*
>
> —Peter Drucker

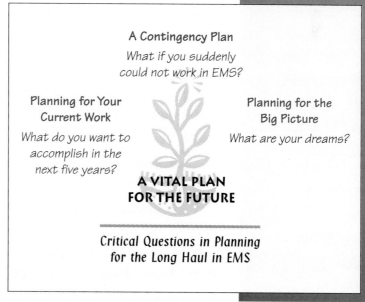

A Contingency Plan
What if you suddenly could not work in EMS?

Planning for Your Current Work
What do you want to accomplish in the next five years?

Planning for the Big Picture
What are your dreams?

A VITAL PLAN FOR THE FUTURE

Critical Questions in Planning for the Long Haul in EMS

fact, many EMS consultants predict that the next ten years will bring unprecedented change in the industry. With the coming of healthcare reform, universal coverage, and managed care systems, EMS systems, organizations, and individual workers will all be affected. No one knows where it will all eventually lead, but there is no question that change is coming, and EMS people need to prepare.

It's hard to say exactly how you should prepare for these changes. In general, EMS leaders agree that the EMS professional of the future must be better educated, more versatile, and more able to adapt to rapid change than ever before.

If you're interested in staying on the street, you may want to begin developing expertise in a relevant area, such as equipment, fleet management, communications, quality, or any other area that you find interesting and that has application to EMS operations. As organizations become more efficient, they will require people who have something unique to offer. Furthermore, don't delay your continuing education. In the coming years, you will likely need an EMS or related degree if you want a good position. You don't need to go to school full-time, but begin taking classes now.

Currently, many EMS professionals are pursuing nursing, physician's assistant, or management degrees. These programs require substantial time to complete and often have waiting lists for entry. By planning now, you can begin to position yourself to realize your plan.

> EMS leaders agree that the EMS professional of the future must be better educated, more versatile, and more able to adapt to rapid change than ever before.

Try This:

Make a five-year plan. Begin by clarifying where you want to be in five years. If this is a foggy area for you, go back to your personal mission statement for EMS and the worksheets from Chapter Three. Consider where you want to be and what the new requirements for your current job might be.

Then complete the following sentence:
In five years, I want to be . . .

_____

_____

Now, think about the accomplishments that will be required during your five-year plan. Break them into five one-year steps.

Year 1	Year 2	Year 3	Year 4	Year 5

The most important part of your plan is getting started; a plan must be worked and revised as it is implemented. It's OK if your plan isn't perfect. Beginning to work on it will make it clear. What can you do this year that will move you toward the five-year mark? What can you do today?

Making a Contingency Plan

Not long ago, a good friend responded to a medical emergency to help an older person who had suffered a stroke. Dana loved working the street and caring for people. She was proud to be a paramedic and had worked hard to earn her position. As she and her partner carried the patient down a flight of stairs, a carpet runner slipped beneath Dana's feet. She stumbled, caught herself, and miraculously hung onto the stretcher. But in that one little move, she twisted her back, and a lumbar disk in her spine ruptured. Pain shot through her back and down her legs.

Somehow, she managed to get the stretcher down the stairs, but it was the last stretcher she would ever carry.

No one plans for a sudden ending to his career, but EMS work is unpredictable, with very real physical demands. Should the time come when you can no longer do the work or are forced by circumstances beyond your control to leave the field, what will you do? Everyone in this work should have a contingency plan for doing something besides EMS. Such a plan helps eliminate the fear of the unknown and can help you prepare for the unexpected. A contingency plan is like having a career insurance policy. It's nice to have just in case.

Think about what you would like to do besides EMS work. At first this may be difficult, but return to your personal mission statement and consider your interests. This plan need not be anything formal or even in writing, but it's something you should begin to think about. Become aware of the many things you could do apart from EMS. What areas of work would appeal to you that have limited physical demands? What preparations can you make now that will prepare you for what lies ahead?

A paramedic named Cindy recently explained why making a contingency plan is so important. On a routine call, she suffered a shoulder injury and found herself unable to return to EMS street work. She had never considered doing anything else, and she had no plan. When she realized she had to consider a different career, she had no idea where to look. A retraining program was available, but in the midst of grieving for her lost career, she couldn't decide what to do.

"Everyone in EMS should be thinking about what they would do if they suddenly had to choose another career," Cindy said. "You can't wait until it happens because in the midst of losing your EMS career, you're so messed up that you can't think with a clear head. You doubt yourself, and you doubt whether you'll ever be fit to do any-

> "Everyone in EMS should be thinking about what they would do if they suddenly had to choose another career."

thing worthwhile again. Even more, though, when you're injured, you're so overwhelmed with your limitations that you can't imagine doing something well again. Everybody should have an idea of what they want to do before something happens."

Successful people do not limit their futures by defining themselves exclusively in terms of a single job. You may be content doing EMS street work, but there are no guarantees of longevity. Preparing yourself for something else frees you to enjoy your work, appreciate its risks, and stop worrying about the unknown.

Planning for the Big Picture

Successful people plan for their immediate future and the unexpected, but they also see the whole of their life and how they want to live. How does EMS fit into your vision of your life? When will you have fulfilled your mission in EMS?

One of the exercises in Chapter Three asked you to make a time line in five-year intervals, beginning at your age now and ending at age 65 or 75. You were encouraged to fill in the things you dreamed about accomplishing in life. What's on your time line? What do you dream about doing in the long run?

Dreams fuel your success. They keep hopes alive, give work purpose, and create anticipation for the future. Often, as we grow older, we stop dreaming; it seems childish. Furthermore, because we may not have realized all of our dreams, we assume that dreams will only set us up for disappointment. But just the opposite is true: If you fail to dream, you will have no future, regardless of your age.

Try This:

Spend some time dreaming. Find a place where you can be by yourself without distractions. With a piece of paper and a

"I'm a paramedic. That's a kind of EMT. I've been promoted to supervisory roles and didn't like them, so I went back to the street. I love it there. My gifts are there. Someday I may die there.

'But what about your career?' my friends ask me.

I say, 'Keep it.'"

—Thom Dick

"Most folks are about as happy as they make up their minds to be."

—Abraham Lincoln

pencil, jot down things you dream about being, doing, and having in your future. Jot down a word or two about each or draw a picture. There's no need to make a list because dreaming isn't linear. Continue until the paper is filled with dreams.

The purpose of this exercise is to help you get in touch with your dreams. If you find dreaming difficult, keep practicing. At first, it will not seem very practical, but as you give yourself permission to dream, you will release the subconscious to begin working on your future and those things you really want from life. All of this relates to your EMS work because you need dreams to help you prepare for the future.

When Is It Time to Quit?

When to leave EMS is always a hotly debated topic among EMS workers. The common opinion says you should leave when you're burned out and frustrated and are providing poor patient care. I disagree. One of the goals of this book is to help you avoid coming to the point where you leave EMS for negative reasons.

People burn out because they lose sight of their purpose, fail to honor themselves, have conflicts with management, or fail to plan their future. If you find yourself frustrated, bored, and cynical about the work, don't just conclude that it's time to quit. Look at your work in terms of the success principles discussed in this book. You'll discover that burnout is not the inevitable end to your EMS work. Rather, burnout is a sign that something is out of balance. Running from EMS may be a temporary fix, but it will not benefit you in the long run. As we mentioned before, creating success today puts us in the best position for success tomorrow.

It's time to leave EMS when you're ready to move on to something else. Instead of running from EMS when it

It's time to leave EMS when you're ready to move on to something else.

gets "too unbearable," move toward your dreams. You'll know it's time to leave when you are excitedly moving toward something new. In order to move toward something new, you will need to be in touch with your dreams and have a plan.

The most frustrated people in EMS work are those who refuse to dream, those for whom EMS work is no longer a challenge and who have nothing to move toward. A common comment is, "I'd like to get out of EMS, but I just don't know what to do." The issue is clearly not the need to leave EMS but the lack of having something to move toward.

Let go of the idea that you'll leave EMS when you're sick of it. Begin by making yourself successful in the work you're doing now, and allow yourself to dream. As you become personally successful in your current EMS work, you'll notice that your entire attitude about staying or leaving is directed by positive rather than negative influences.

Rewarding Yourself

People who create success in EMS not only plan for the future, but also reward themselves. EMS workers often wait in vain for supervisors, managers, and the community to recognize their contributions. Unfortunately, much of EMS work does not attract attention. Occasionally EMS workers will respond to the scene of a well-publicized disaster or rescue in which they are recognized for their contributions, but most of what EMS workers do is done quietly. You will not be openly rewarded for the extra comfort you give that nursing home patient. There will be no parades for the times you go the extra mile in caring for someone.

EMS remains a profession that receives very little recognition. You may work for low pay and few benefits and often without any sort of future retirement or "reward" at the end of your service. It becomes easy to tell yourself

People who create success in EMS not only plan for the future, but also reward themselves.

that the work doesn't matter. Therefore, it is imperative that you reward yourself.

This may sound silly. How do you reward yourself? Do you organize an award ceremony for one? Do you strain the muscles in your upper arm patting yourself on the back? Not exactly. But you must recognize and honor your own achievements.

After completing a consulting project for a large ALS service, I stopped by the house of one of the paramedic supervisors. He has been in EMS for several years and is one of the most personally successful people in EMS that I know. He is well respected by his employees and has a healthy, relaxed attitude about his position. One entire wall of his den is covered with EMS patches, pictures, and certificates. "What's all this?" I asked. "That's my wall of fame," he said, smiling and turning on several track lights that illuminated the wall. "It's my own personal EMS hall of fame."

The wall is his way of acknowledging and honoring his achievements in the field. It holds news clippings of calls he's been on, training certificates, and pictures of co-workers. He is immensely proud of this personal hall of fame.

"During my first month on the street, I went to a bad call, a house fire where an older couple died," he explained, pointing to a faded yellow newspaper clipping. "We worked on this couple—it was my first arrest, a double arrest—but we couldn't save them, so no one really paid any attention to how hard we had worked or that it was my first big call and first contact with death. I waited and waited for my boss, or medical director, or someone to say something about the call, but no one did. I felt like I needed to do something, so I cut out the articles and stuck them on the wall, and it made me feel a lot better. Anyway, I just keep sticking up stuff. I'm pretty proud of what I do."

You must recognize and honor your own achievements.

This paramedic discovered something very important: While helping people has its own intrinsic rewards, you still need to acknowledge and honor your accomplishments in EMS work. For you, it may not be a wall of fame or a scrapbook; it may be treating yourself well when you've had a good or bad shift and done the right thing.

It's easy to diminish the fact that you worked a shift in which you cared for a man with an MI, successfully treated an asthma victim, and transported a young woman who was threatening to kill herself. But all of these are important achievements worthy of reward. How do you treat yourself after a shift? Do you take time to do something nurturing and rewarding?

You should reward yourself in the same way you would reward someone else. Acknowledge that an important thing has been done, and then do something nice for yourself. Sitting down and eating a leisurely meal, taking yourself out for a special treat, or in some way acknowledging yourself with something you value is how you reward yourself. Creating enduring success has little to do with climbing ladders or big, grand achievements. Creating success will continue to be about your personal relationship with the work and how you value what you do.

Muddy Roads

Have you noticed how things always seem to go wrong during a multiple casualty incident?. Whether it's a drill or a real incident, it always seems as if something goes awry—a missed radio signal, confusion at the command post, or an unforeseen twist, such as hazardous materials or a fire. Suddenly the neat disaster plan is completely off track. The same thing happens in creating personal success in your career. Success doesn't mean everything will go smoothly.

There will be periods when you become frustrated with

"I do not happen to be a believer in the cliché, 'Virtue is its own reward.' As far as I'm concerned, the reward for virtue should be at least a chocolate sundae, and preferably a cruise to the Bahamas."

—Barbara Sher

"The reward, the real grace, of conscious service . . . is the opportunity not only to help relieve suffering but to grow in wisdom, experience greater unity, and have a good time while we're doing it."

—Ram Dass

the work, when the job appears to be a dead end, and when you become weary of shifts and the limited sense of accomplishment. Furthermore, your life is much more than EMS—a divorce, a death in the family, a personal awakening, financial problems, or even a period of personal neglect may all be part of life's journey and can send you into a muddy part of the road where success seems impossible.

Several years ago, in trying to do everything at once and have it all, I found both my professional and personal life deeply mired in mud. I halfheartedly shuffled through a few EMS jobs, not doing any of them well. I went through a difficult divorce and for a period of time found myself completely without direction. I did not feel as if I was creating success, and rather than coming together, everything seemed to be falling apart.

It is human nature to view life in terms of current events. If something is going badly, we have a tendency to assess our entire lives—or at least the immediate future—negatively. Yet consider what happens in the MCI drill. No matter what goes wrong and how many setbacks occur, you simply continue on. Somehow, it works out. The hazards are managed, the patients are treated and transported, and the entire experience is educational. The unpredictable happenings and the muddy parts of the road often teach the most.

I discovered that mistakes were not the end of my success. I also discovered that both successful and unsuccessful people become stuck in the mud. The difference is, successful people don't give up. They keep trying. The writer Richard Bach says, "There are no mistakes. The events we bring upon ourselves, no matter how unpleasant, are necessary in order to learn what we need to learn; whatever steps we take, they're necessary to reach the places we've chosen to go."

These difficult times signal the beginning of growth

Successful people don't give up.

and forward movement. If you find yourself stuck, far from feeling successful and far from where you hoped to be, don't let despair lead you. With the perspective of time, you'll discover you are doing better than you think.

Ultimate Success

Hopefully, you have found much in this book that will be useful in creating your success in EMS. Hopefully, you have realized that success is unique to who you are and what you want from your EMS experience. As you can see, there is no single path to success or secret formula that will magically make your EMS work satisfying and meaningful.

Yet, EMS itself is a very special place to begin creating success in more than just your job. EMS is a spiritual work. It allows you to touch again and again the mysteries of birth, life, death, human suffering, and compassion. But even more than that, your daily EMS work gives you a unique opportunity to practice the universal truth of all religions—that it is more blessed to give than to receive.

The American philosopher and writer Ralph Waldo Emerson said, "It is one of the most beautiful compensations of this life that no man can sincerely try to help another without helping himself."

As I write this, it is early morning, and I have just completed a long, busy night shift. There were several calls—a drunk driver who ran into a utility pole, a middle-aged woman with chronic back pain, and finally, early this morning just before the end of the shift, an elderly man with congestive heart failure. I'm tired, but I also have a powerful sense of success. I did not change the world during my night shift nor did I save a life; but I was able to make a contribution to my world through my work while also contributing to my own success.

EMS is full of spiritual wealth and opportunity. You

EMS is a spiritual work. It allows you to touch again and again the mysteries of birth, life, death, human suffering, and compassion.

may not become rich by society's standards, but as you learn to create your success, you'll discover that EMS is indeed full of unlimited richness.

Good luck.

Summary

✔ A growing number of people are creating lasting success in EMS without burning out.

✔ The characteristics of people who create long-term success in EMS are

1) They love what they do.

2) They monitor the amount of time they work and continue to grow.

3) They have a vital plan for their future.

✔ To plan for your future in EMS, you must

1) Make a specific plan for the next five years.

2) Make a contingency plan in case your EMS work is interrupted.

3) Continue to dream and keep the whole of your life in mind.

✔ It's time to leave EMS work when you are ready to move on to something else.

✔ Staying happy in EMS work demands that you learn to reward yourself.

✔ The muddy roads along your success journey need not stop you—they are part of the process.

✔ The ultimate success in EMS comes as you begin to realize the richness of your work.

Suggested Reading

Living Happily Ever After: Creating Trust, Luck, and Joy, by Marsha Sinetar (Villard Books, New York, 1990). One of the lessons of EMS is that nothing remains the same. Security is an illusion. This book is about finding success and happiness in the midst of change and adversity.

Mid-Career Crisis, by Jean Russell Nave and Louise M. Nelson (Perigee Books, New York, 1991). What happens when in the midst of your career you decide you want to do something else? How can you move from one thing to another and still keep your sanity? This is a great guide book from people who have done it.

The Overworked American: The Unexpected Decline of Leisure, by Juliet B. Schor (Harper Collins, New York, 1991). Do you feel like you're working more than ever? You probably are, and here's the proof. The author provides a startling look at how much we really work and some of the effects overwork is having on us and on our society.

Take this Job and Love It: A Personal Guide to Career Empowerment, by Diane Tracy (McGraw-Hill, New York, 1994). Do you feel trapped in your work setting? Has the fun gone out of your EMS work? Learn how to practice the principle of "loving what you do."

When All You've Ever Wanted Isn't Enough, by Harold Kushner (Pocket Books, New York, 1986). This must-read book is about how to be successful in life. It is about creating a life that is worth living and finding contentment and peace in the long haul.

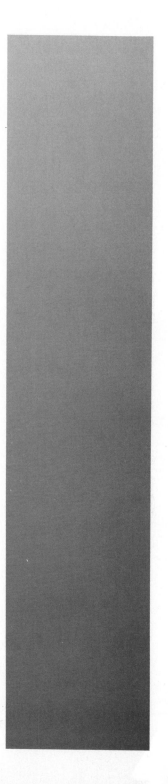

About the Author

John Becknell is a writer, consultant, and paramedic from Minnesota. He began his work in EMS in 1975 and has worked as an EMT, paramedic, flight medic, instructor, and consultant. He has also worked on international EMS development projects in the Middle East and Central America. John's writing often appears in the *Journal of Emergency Medical Services (JEMS)*, where he is known for writing about the non-technical side of EMS work. Currently, he provides motivational and professional development seminars for EMS workers throughout the country and continues to work as a paramedic at Ridgeview Medical Center in Waconia, Minnesota.